Apple Cider Vinegar

Enjoy the Whole Benefits of Apple Cider Vinegar

(Health Benefits and Healing Powers of Apple Cider Vinegar)

Jeffrey Ramirez

Published By **Tyson Maxwell**

Jeffrey Ramirez

Apple Cider Vinegar: Enjoy the Whole Benefits of Apple Cider Vinegar (Health Benefits and Healing Powers of Apple Cider Vinegar)

ISBN 978-1-77485-766-3

No part of this guidebook shall be reproduced in any form without permission in writing from the publisher except in the case of brief quotations embodied in critical articles or reviews.

Legal & Disclaimer

The information contained in this ebook is not designed to replace or take the place of any form of medicine or professional medical advice. The information in this ebook has been provided for educational & entertainment purposes only.

The information contained in this book has been compiled from sources deemed reliable, and it is accurate to the best of the Author's knowledge; however, the Author cannot guarantee its accuracy and validity and cannot be held liable for any errors or omissions. Changes are periodically made to this book. You must consult your doctor or get professional medical advice before using any of the suggested remedies, techniques, or information in this book.

Upon using the information contained in this book, you agree to hold harmless the Author from and against any damages, costs, and expenses, including any legal fees potentially resulting from the application of any of the information provided by this guide. This disclaimer applies to any damages or injury caused by the use and application, whether directly or indirectly, of any advice or information presented, whether for breach of contract, tort, negligence, personal injury, criminal intent, or under any other cause of action.

You agree to accept all risks of using the information presented inside this book. You need to consult a professional medical practitioner in order to ensure you are both able and healthy enough to participate in this program.

TABLE OF CONTENTS

Introduction

Apple cider vinegar may be the most effective natural remedy documented throughout the history of mankind. Its use as a remedy has been documented as early as 5500 BC from the Babylonians who utilized the date palm for making vinegar and wine.

It was used to make food as well as picking agents. Vinegar remnants have been discovered in the oldest Egyptian Urns dating back to 3000 BC. Chinese historical documents dating to 1200 BC extol the greatness of vinegar's benefits too.

The motives behind its widespread medical use as well as as an energy drink have been scientifically supported by the latest science. Apple cider vinegar's benefits result from its origin - the noble apple, which is popular for its saying that an apple daily keeps the doctor at bay.

Apples are packed with vitamins, antioxidants, minerals, but also the dietary fiber. Additionally, they contain no sodium or fat.

The apple's goodness is magically transferred into cider vinegar made from apple, particularly when it's left untreated or, in other words, not processed.

Apple cider vinegar made of whole apples, not processed or pasteurized includes not just all of the apple's nutrients, but also numerous other organic acids and enzymes that are created by the two fermentations needed to convert apples into vinegar.

The many benefits from apple cider can range from antiseptic to antioxidant. It also provides a range of minerals that are absorbable, such as magnesium and potassium as well as pectin. It also contains water-soluble fiber, which is among the numerous reasons behind the effectiveness in the diet of cider vinegar.

The most effective method for using Apple cider vinegar would be to transform it into a tonic making a mixture of 2 or 3 teaspoons ACV into an 8-ounce glass of water. You can drink it prior to or after every meal.

A key thing to keep in mind when you are taking apple cider vinegar after meals or prior to sleeping is to clean your mouth in order to prevent the long-term contact of vinegar with your enamel teeth.

Another method of tackling this minor inconvenience is to mix 1 tsp. of baking soda into the vinegar prior to adding water. It's always enjoyable to watch it bubble up! In addition to the alkalinity added by baking soda is definitely a health benefit.

When ACV solutions are concerned, the list is literally From A-Z. It begins with asthma and acne, and then progresses to warts , weight loss and warts and ends with yeast infections, including diseases like cancer, eczemaand fatigue and headaches. insomnia, heartburn ulcers, sore throat and varicose veins between, to name just the most common.

In the end the apple cider vinegar does not disappoint in its claim as being the most straightforward solution to a perfect health, and a long-lasting cure too. A must-have in any natural medicine cabinet and a potent preventative for any ailment, and not to forget its old-fashioned fame as a world-class tonic.

Always use organic, unprocessed apple cider vinegar that has the mother still present and you can count on its incredible qualities to ensure that your family and you with a long, healthy life.

This GUIDE is fully packed with all the wonders ACV offers.

Let's dive in!

Chapter 1: Is A Great Drink For Your Health

We all know the old saying: an apple every day helps keep doctors away. Apples can be made into a vinegar type. Many studies have proven the amazing benefits of apple cider vinegar.

While they were known before however, the advantages were not recognized as significant. A lot of people only think of it as a cooking condiment.

You may have seen numerous books that highlight the many advantages that apple cider vinegar has to offer. What exactly is vinegar, and why can it benefit you? It is created by crushing apples to make a mixture of pulp and juices; the mixture is allowed to ferment for a while until Acetic acid is created.

One of the most popular applications for this rich vinegar-based supplement is weight loss. Many people claim that they easily lose weight simply by drinking 2 tablespoons of the nectar every day and each day. This is the sole condition for your diet. Simply take the vinegar and you'll be getting closer to slimmer and healthier.

It is not clear on how it can aid in weight loss However, people who have used this vinegar report they lost the weight of a significant amount which they believe was due to the normal drinking of vinegar.

It is widely thought that the minerals, vitamins amino acids, amino acids and enzymes enhance our metabolism at same time that they reduce appetite naturally. This is why the efficacy of apple cider in weight loss was widely recognized.

It is feasible to make use of the apple cider vinegar for home remedies for many ailments. A popular theory is its anti-aging properties. It is able to perform cleansing and detoxification functionsthat result in the body's detoxification.

As a healing potion, it is a natural antibiotic and antiseptics, which are used by the body in order to fight bacteria and germs in the human body, specifically in digestion. It also aids the digestive system because it breaks down nutrients, proteins, fats, and minerals in the food you consume.

It is possible to earn the benefits of apple cider vinegar when you consume it every day. You can use it for dressing salads or marinade. It can also be purchased in capsules. If you're looking to make your own apple cider vinegar you'll discover several things you need be aware of so that the vinegar can be beneficial.

There are numerous steps you must be following, and you should avoid using metal containers or aluminum. You can make this mix using glass wood, plastic enamel, stainless steel and other materials. It is essential to keep an eye out on completing each step, which includes fermentation to make vinegar with success.

Chapter 2: Health Benefits Of Apple Cider Vinegar

The apple cider vinegar (ACV) is often referred to as an all-purpose cure for anything. People who are health conscious have used it to treat everything from allergies and acne to warts, sore throats, and sore throats. Vinegar in its various variants has been used over ages for all kinds of remedies from folklore.

In recent times, with the influx of individuals turning towards home remedies and natural remedies Apple cider vinegar has been uncovered as a highly effective supplement to health.

There is a lot of doubt about an item as basic like apple cider vinegar, which is an effective remedy for many illnesses. Traditional healers have for a long time utilized apple cider vinegar as a natural remedy for many ailments.

If you think of apple cider, you likely picture the fall. A warm, sweet glass of spice and apples that warms your body on a cold autumn day. This delicious drink is where this amazing tonic starts.

It is born as apples which are crushed into cider. This cider is then infused with yeast, which transforms the sugars contained in it into alcohol. At this point the is fermented until the wine becomes sour and then turns into vinegar.

ACV has numerous claims to fame. Some of them include:

A natural acne reducing agent and toner for the skin.

* A wart remover

* A hair wash to refresh and nourish dull hair.

* Get rid of ticks, fleas, lice and more

* Cure infections

* Eliminates the toxins

* A natural aftershave

* Reduces the risk of sunburn.

* And much more!

The main advantages of apple cider vinegar is the positive effects that occur inside the body. If you add it to your diet daily the effects are impressive. Let's examine some of these advantages:

Increased Digestion and Weight Loss

ACV can assist in restoring normal levels of acid in your digestive system , which assists in breaking down fats as well as proteins. This helps your body digest food faster and more efficiently, which improves absorption of nutrients by your body and overall general health.

Apple cider vinegar may also aid in feeling fuller, and aid in reducing your appetite and ease some of the burden off the digestive tract.

It has also been proven to regulate blood sugar levels, which aids in weight loss and reduces the risk of developing diabetes. A study also found that regular consumption of apple cider vinegar decreased body fat and the levels of triglycerides and helped with general weight loss. It's an excellent weight loss supplement , and is a simple way to tackle weight gain.

Aids in Preventing Cancer

Apple cider vinegar reduces the growth of cancerous cells, and may even kill cancer cells. The findings of research have not been entirely reliable regarding this topic, however there are many possibilities. Many believe that the acetic acid found in vinegar is a anti-cancer ingredient.

Some have suggested the pectin in apples and polyphenols as potential anti-cancer ingredients. The source of the ingredient is unknown, but preliminary evidence suggests the apple cider vinegar can be effective in the fight against certain forms of cancer.

Increased Cholesterol Levels and Blood Pressure

A preliminary study conducted on rats has demonstrated the fact that vinegar made from apple has the ability to dramatically reduce cholesterol levels within the body. Since the research was done on rats, many speculate that the properties might not be as effective in humans. More research is needed to confirm this, however preliminary evidence suggests that it is.

Similar studies also demonstrated positive results in the reduction of the blood pressure as well as heart disease. Due to the low amount of adverse effects as well as evidence that suggests it can reduce the risk factors overall for heart disease, taking a regular intake in apple cider vinegar could be an ideal suggestion.

The Liver as well as Other Organs Detoxification

The antibacterial qualities that apple cider vinegar has assist to rid the body of toxins buildup and decrease the amount of bacteria that cause harm. Your body's PH equilibrium is maintained through regular dosages, which assists in the natural cleansing effects of the body.

It has been utilized to treat allergies too by flushing mucous out of the sinuses and cleaning the lymph nodes.

If you are considering drinking apple cider vinegar ensure you get unfiltered, organic, or unpasteurized, vinegar. Vinegar that is not treated will enhance the health benefits.

Before you begin any supplementation regimen or even one that is organic, talk with your physician about potential negative interactions and effects with other medicines you're taking. Apple cider vinegar is available straight from the bottle , or in other forms like pills to reduce the sour flavor and acidity.

Chapter 3: How To Use Apple Cider Vinegar For Weight Loss

The vinegar of apple cider is produced through the fermentation of apple juice. It's a natural treatment for a range of ailments and has been used for many years.

It has lots to offer in regards to weight loss. It assists to break down complex carbohydrates and fats and lowers blood sugar levels and cholesterol levels; lessens hunger cravings and aids in digestion and detoxification of the body.

It is a natural, low-calorie supplement that contains a variety of nutrients and active ingredients - minerals Vitamins, soluble fibers, vitamins antioxidants, enzymes and natural acids that help fight the problem of obesity.

It is essential to understand the fact that concentrated apple cider vinegar (undiluted) in its undiluted form, is a very strong acid that shouldn't be consumed in its raw form. The Esophagus Tube (food pipe) isn't equipped to handle it and may be damaged severely.

Therefore, it is sensible to dilute the dosage by adding water to ensure that the intensity is reduced. Additionally, it is essential to keep track of the dosage frequently. Begin with 5-10 milliliters daily, and gradually increase it to

30ml (2 tablespoons) each day. The amount that is higher than 30 milliliters is usually not recommended.

Let's talk about the ways Apple Cider Vinegar will help you shed some pounds and make a change in your life positive:

* Aids in reducing Cholesterol levels

Bile is a viscous yellowish fluid produced by the liver. It assists to break down diet-related fats and also to eliminate away cholesterol as well as other toxins from the liver. Insufficient bile production can hinder liver's activity, which can result in the accumulation of cholesterol and fats that result in weight gain.

Consuming one tablespoon apple cider vinegar in the early hours of the morning can kick-start production of bile to aid in the breakdown of fat and cholesterol.

* Lowers blood sugar levels.

A rise in blood sugar levels can trigger cravings for snacks and processed foods , which is an irritant for those trying to lose some weight.

* Helps block Carbohydrates (starch)

There is no longer a time where it was thought that carbohydrates are harmful to health.

Dieticians in the new age recommends that you consume carbohydrates regularly to maintain a balanced diet.

The starch found in carbohydrates tends to convert quickly into glucose and increase an insulin release into the body. The insulin stimulates an accumulation of glucose as fat. Therefore, eating foods that are starchy can trigger your body into energy storage phase.

How can Apple Cider Vinegar going to benefit us?

The amount of acetic acid in the vinegar affects digestion of starch by the human body. It aids in reducing the storage of glucose as fat. In the long run the starch blockage process is sure to have an impact on weight of the body.

* Supports the health of your digestive system

The gut is home to trillions of probiotics (healthy bacteria) which help break down the food particles complex to fight the growth of microbes that cause disease and regulate the immune system.

Apple cider vinegar serves as a catalyst to these probiotics. Probiotics feed off the pectins within apple cider vinegar to aid expansion and growth. Thus apple cider vinegar aids to maintain a healthy gut flora to ensure a healthy digestive system and metabolism.

* Reduces appetite

Pectins are the main ingredient in apple cider vinegarwhich are soluble fibers that provide an impression of fullness and helps curb appetite, for all the best reasons.

* It functions as diuretic and mild laxative in nature.

Apple cider vinegar is an effective mild laxative that can speed up the elimination process, and also ensure regular elimination and regular bowel movement. Additionally, it provides an effect that diuresis to flush out the water stored in the body.

* Promote body detox

Body detoxification is the comprehensive elimination of the body to rid the body of all accumulated wastes- food particles that are not digested cholesterol, saturated fats, cholesterol and disease-causing microbes. Because of a poor eating habits and poor lifestyle the body's metabolism begins to slow and the accumulation of body toxins begins.

The combination of slow body metabolism and the accumulation of toxic substances in the body can lead to weight gain. It is an apple cider vinegar cleansing drink that is natural and safe. It helps to improve digestion, speed the metabolism of your body helps relieve constipation, and eliminates excess water out of your body. This helps detoxify your body's internal organs.

How to consume Apple Cider Vinegar

Mix 1-2 teaspoons (5-10 milliliters) of apple cider vinegar into one glass (250 milliliters) of water. Stir well before drinking it prior to meals. If it causes a temporary irritation or heartburn, you can dilute it by adding more water. It can be mixed with juice or other drinks too. Some people like to sprinkle it on salads or other food items according to their preference.

The recommended dosage for a day is 30 milliliters.

Safety measures and potential adverse consequences

In general the case, Apple cider vinegar can be described as a healthy drink that is safe for anyone of any age. Be aware of the following safety guidelines to reap the maximum advantages:

Do not drink it the first thing in the morning - empty stomach, as it can irritate your gut liner and trigger a burning sensation.

* Mix it with enough water1 teaspoon into one glass of water is a acceptable proportion.

*Due to the acidity, excessive drinking of vinegar made from apple could harm the esophagus and tissues. It can also cause hypokalemia, which is condition where the amount of potassium levels in blood drop below the level required.

Make sure to wash your mouth thoroughly after drinking apple cider vinegar, as the acidity in vinegar could cause abrasion to tooth enamel. It can also cause yellow staining on your teeth.

* In the first few days following the consumption it is possible to experience short-term symptoms like stomach cramps, diarrhea and heartburn, or headache. In the majority of cases the symptoms will fade disappear within a couple of days. If they persist then stop taking the medication and talk to a medical professional

* Women who are pregnant, nursing women, and those suffering from chronic health issues

should consult their physician prior to taking this.

Start slowlystarting with a small amount, and gradually increase the amount to 2 tablespoons per day in a properly diluted form for the best outcomes.

The benefits from apple cider vinegar in weight loss are evident. However, as an all-natural remedy, it shouldn't be considered the ultimate cure and would produce the best results if used in conjunction with a balanced low-calorie diet, a healthy life style that includes regular exercise.

Chapter 4: Apple Cider Vinegar Flu Remedy

It has been utilized to cure a variety of diseases over the years. If one can overcome its unpleasant taste, there is relief from its healing qualities.

One of its most common reasons is to ward off the flu or cold. It's believed to help alleviate a sore throat help ease a recurring cough and treat sinus infections and the typical symptoms of an illness like a cold or flu. Making use of apple cider vinegar as a flu treatment is simple and natural. It is also safe for most people.

How does it work

If you get an illness, your body's pH level becomes more alkaline. Apple cider vinegar which is acidic aids in balancing your body's acidity.

Sinus Infection

If you have an infection of the sinus In the event of a sinus infection, the apple cider vinegar cure can reduce the production of mucus and can eliminate watery eyes due to its large quantities of potassium.

It can rapidly thin the mucous and turn it from thick green to translucent to white, and fluid. Apple cider vinegar is a rich source of nutrients, vitamins, and trace elements like iron, copper silica magnesium, phosphorous and calcium.

How do you take it

There are a variety of ways to incorporate the apple cider vinegar in your daily diet to reap its beneficial effects. The effectiveness of an apple cider vinegar-based flu remedy isn't solely dependent on the method you use to take this remedy. It also relies how often you consume it. Some people use it as a daily remedy or drink, while others consume it right at the first indication of sinus or cold inflammation.

Since it has a bitter taste It is usually blended with different liquids. You can dilute 1/8 - 1 cup apple cider vinegar in 16 8 ounces of juice or water and drink it all day long.

If you're the adventurous kind, mix two tablespoons apple cider vinegar in 8 glasses of water or juice and then drink the entire mixture in one go, three times a every day.

If it is added to cider, the drink tasted like cider, and is more refreshing to drink.

It is also possible to stir it in a tea cup.

In the event that drinking vinegar from apple cider isn't in the question, then add it to marinades, sauces, or dressings.

The dosage recommended to take apple cider vinegar amounts as high as 3 tablespoons per day. It's also sold in capsules at a variety of vitamin and health food stores. A daily dose of a capsule helps keep your body's pH steady, making you immune systems strong enough to combat colds and flu.

Other Alternative Remedial Uses in Apple Cider Vinegar for Flu

For help in easing chest congestion caused by the flu or cold, wash a small piece of brown newspaper in apple cider vinegar. Then place it on one side of black pepper. The paper should be secured (pepper-side down) over the chest and allow it to sit for around 30 minutes.

To ease a snoring cough that is caused by the flu or cold, sprinkle apple cider vinegar on the pillows before you go to sleep.

To ease the pain of a throat caused by the flu or cold mix equal parts of vinegar made from apple cider and warm water. gargle regularly, making sure you rinse your mouth well afterward to stop acid from destroying the enamel of your teeth.

To ease a headache due to sinus and nasal congestion Add 1/8 cup of apple cider vinegar into the solution of water inside the vaporizer.

Chapter 5: Apple Cider Vinegar Benefits For Beauty

Apple cider vinegar also called ACV or cider vinegar, is made from apple or cider must. It is now very well-known due to its many health benefits and cosmetic properties.

Because of its potassium content, it's advised to consult an expert in health before using ACV. While Apple cider vinegar can be made at home, it's possible to buy it in its natural form in any health food retailer. Let's look at some of the advantages from apple cider vinegar.

How to make use of apple cider vinegar?

Apple cider vinegar is a great way to aid in promoting healthier hair and skin and can be beneficial for your health. To learn more about the ways that apple cider vinegar can aid in treating specific illnesses, speak to an expert in nutrition who is more knowledgeable to address specific questions. For general applications you can test apples cider vinegar any of the below ways.

Internal use

Studies have shown that ACV aids the body in its everyday tasks as well as fighting against colds and flu. It helps with digestion, reduces bad cholesterol it strengthens the heart, reduces blood pressure, and helps stabilize blood sugar levels. It also contains antioxidants that aid in fighting certain types of cancer. It is a remedy for digestive upset by taking it regularly as a tonic.

For your own homemade drink, combine equal amounts of honey and apple cider vinegar in the glass of water. Typically, 1 teaspoon ACV as well as 1 tablespoon of honey mixed in 8 ounces of warm or cold water will be a reasonable guideline However, you are at liberty to modify the recipe based on your individual preferences.

There are different methods to consume it. You can mix it with apple juice, or add some fresh cinnamon to balance the taste (some cafes serve apple cider with cinnamon sticks).

External use

If your feet are exhausted and painful you should bathe them. Add half a cup apple cider vinegar into the tub with warm water. Relax your feet and allow your feet to soak for several minutes. A footbath can be a wonderful opportunity to relax before settling down to sleep.

When your body's pH is acidic, you can take the vinegar bath. In order to restore the acid-alkaline balance within your body, just include 1 to 2 cups apple cider vinegar into an ice bath. The body will be soaked for approximately 45 minutes. Apart from cleansing your body of acid, a bath in vinegar aids anyone with rough or dry skin to create a soft and smooth feeling.

If baths aren't your style take a look at mixing one cup of warm and ACV into the spray bottle. After you shower you can sprinkle your entire body with the mix. After a few minutes, wash. Your entire body will feel rejuvenated.

Other advantages other benefits of using apple cider vinegar comprise its use for various body parts, particularly the face. For a deeply cleansing steam face wash make sure you add three tablespoons ACV in boiling water in a pan and place your face in it.

Protect your hair with towels for a couple of minutes to let the steam make your pores more open and remove any impurities that may be on the skin's surface.

Commercial products available on the market

Apart from the natural form from apple cider vinegar a variety of commercial products are also available. These include body washes, products for facial and hair. It is important to note that ACV as it is can be just as effective, if not more than the products.

Since the apple cider vinegar can be highly acidic, you should never consume it in one go. Always dilute it by adding water. After drinking ACV then you must wash your mouth using water. Do not floss your teeth as soon as you finish since it may make the vinegar abrasive to your enamel.

An excellent way to keep ACV from touching your teeth drinking it through straws. ACV tablets are an excellent alternative to the liquid however they aren't as quickly. Avoid contact with the eyes using apple cider vinegar because the acid can cause burning and cause redness to the eyes.

The advantages that apple cider vinegar can provide are to be endless. The easy methods and ways of making use of ACV are all fantastic and affordable. In addition, they offer proved methods that are that are beneficial for your body and to the planet. If you utilize it in a controlled manner and for recognized beneficial purposes, the Apple cider vinegar's benefits are bound to continue to show their benefits.

Chapter 6: How To Use Apple Cider Vinegar To Cure Acne

Apple Cider Vinegar otherwise known as (ACV) is a powerful natural antibiotic with numerous elements like magnesium, calcium, potassium and sodium. It also contains chlorine iron, sulfur, many more.

These elements are all essential to a healthy body, especially for promoting the development of healthy skin. This anti-bacterial property makes it an excellent home-based solution for acne.

The principal ingredient in ACV is Acetic acid. It aids in exfoliating dead skin cells, gently. It also eliminates the propionibacterium acnes bacteria commonly referred to as P-acnes. It neutralizes sebum, which is the oily substance P-acnes feeds upon and thrives on.

How do you make Apple Cider Vinegar produced?

It is produced through the fermentation process of apple cider, or apple must, which is made from organically crushed apples. To clarify fermentation is a process of transformation.

Organic apples have a certain amount of yeast and bacteria in their peels. Therefore, when you crush them, you'll get pure apple juice, which is the combination of yeast and bacteria.

Then you let it to mature for a time. The sugar present in this cider breaks into smaller pieces by bacteria and yeast, which transforms into alcohol. It's more of an brewing process that eventually transforms into vinegar following another fermentation.

If you're not able to find the time or the resources to create one at home, you can buy ACV from any of the departmental store. The first thing to do is ensure you purchase organic ACV that has the label with the words "With the Mother" with an acidity (pH) range between five and seven.

It is in pure and raw form. It is characterized by dark cloudy web-like bacterial foam, which is brownish in hue.

The benefits of Vinegar Apple Cider Your Skin

ACV has acids, among them is alpha-hydroxy acid, which has taken directly from apples. These acids aid in dissolving the sebum and oil which clogs pores, and then clear them. This can encourage the renewal of skin.

It is believed to help treat allergies from food, pets and environmental pollutants, as well as flu, high cholesterol, sinus infections, chronic fatigue and sore throats. It also helps with arthritis and gout , to mention some.

The most well-known benefit is linked to weight reduction. ACV is believed to reduce fat and that a regular dose of vinegar from apple cider mixed into water aids in keeping the blood pressure of high patients under the control of just two weeks.

It also aids in regulating the acidity of the face by diluting it using two parts of water before applying the mixture to your face with an old cotton ball to act as an overnight toner and washing it off in the following morning. Make sure you dilute it using larger amounts of water because you will be leaving the product all over your body for a number of days.

It also assists in reducing age spots by applying ACV directly onto them for around 20 minutes or so per day, depending on the size. Additionally, it can help cleanse your liver by ridding it of toxins that have accumulated and recharge its effectiveness.

How do you apply Apple Cider Vinegar for acne?

The application of this is dependent according to the degree of acne. The majority of users dilute it with some water and apply it using the help of a cotton ball on their acne spots, as it appears to be effective. ACV is considered to be a suitable alternative to antibiotics because it aids in treating bacteria that cause infections.

It is possible to make use of cider vinegar apple cider in two different ways: one is as an internal tonic and as a topical antibacterial remedy.

Following these instructions, you could be able to see impressive outcomes. Take three tablespoons of ACV into the bottle of water, and mix them well. Then , apply it to your face using the help of a cotton ball to act to act as an Astringent.

Try 3 different types of cotton balls to massage your face. You can use one on your forehead, one for your nose and cheeks, and the third one for your cheeks. If you have an oily nose then use a different one to treat that.

This prevents the spread of bacteria from one spot across your face, which could lead to more breakouts in other parts of the face. While this isn't a huge problem but it's always better to be secure rather than regretting it.

Let it sit for 10 to fifteen minutes , then rinse it off thoroughly using warm water. Use a soft, cloth to rub the skin dry. Repeat this process 3 times per day to get the best results.

If you suffer from severe acne infections You can apply a smaller doses of ACV dilute with 3 to 4 parts of water. You can leave it overnight to complete its job . Then rinse it off the next day using warm water.

Make sure you apply a less strength ACV if you decide to apply it to your skin and allow it to remain the skin on for extended time.

Another way to use it is drink it with water and a couple of tablespoons of table spoons to drink as an all-day tonic. It helps stop acne breakouts, decrease inflammation, and also dry out the inflammation. The only thing keep in mind is the fact that it may not taste very pleasant. You can drink it as water and you'll be good to go.

If you're dealing with painful pimples that are prominent I suggest mixing one tablespoon of ACV and three parts of water , and rub it on the pimple. It should remain there for around 15 minutes before washing it off using warm water.

A few Tips and Warns

Don't apply full strength ACV to the face because there are reports of irritations, skin damage and burns. Therefore, be cautious when applying this treatment, especially for those with sensitive skin.

Always use unfiltered, raw as well as unpasteurized cider vinegar. This will yield the most efficient outcomes.

After applying Apple cider vinegar rub tea tree oil onto your acne. Tea tree oil works wonders for healing skin.

If you're allergic to apples and apple cider vinegar, apple cider vinegar may not the right choice for you.

Do not mix it with other acne medication. This can cause problems and dryness of the skin.

When applying ACV It is recommended to begin by using the simplest mixture comprising four parts water to it. If you're confident with it, move on to stronger combinations. This means that you have to reduce amounts of water.

Tingling sensations are normal with ACV however, when you begin to feel burning sensations, you should wash the area immediately with cold water.

Apple cider vinegar in general is generally positive with the exception of the astringency of the vinegar, which you should be wary of using on your face. I suggest beginning with a lower amount of it, and gradually increasing the strength to a higher level as you become more accustomed to the solution for your skin.

It's normal to experience a discomfort as it's an indication of the fact that it's functioning. If you notice burning symptoms, take it off right away and decrease the strength of ACV.

For best results, you should use an oil-based moisturizer for your skin for your skin following each ACV treatment. This helps to keep your skin from becoming dry due to the astringent properties of ACV.

I'd want to emphasize that, even though apple cider vinegar is able to eliminate some bacteria that are present on the skin, it's not a solution for long-term use that is able to tackle acne from the root. There are many reasons for acne and bacteria is one of them.

It's better or worse for people with moderate to mild acne. You may see results within few weeks. If you have severe acne it may take several months to heal. Keep your eyes open and you'll dominate the world! The best part is that you're doing it naturally and certainly not burning your wallet while doing it.

It's logical to test this low-cost DIY remedy before committing to more expensive treatments. If you do need to go to the doctor, the extent of your acne could have been reduced and you would not have to wait for a long time going through any medical procedure prescribed with any dermatologist.

Chapter 7: Get Rid Of Dandruff With Apple Cider Vinegar

If you're suffering from dandruff, then you are aware of how irritating and itchy this condition can be. It might feel as if there's no solution that can help with dandruff, but you've attempted to find it. What if the answer was not in the medication aisle?

In reality, it could be on the shelves of your local grocery store. It is possible to get rid of hair flakes with apples cider vinegar. It's possible that you're wondering what acidity can be applied to your scalp. If you're exhausted of the itching, get rid of itchy scalp with Apple cider vinegar.

Dandruff are white flakes of hair that can be that are found over the head. It rarely causes any other issues besides the discomforting itching. There are many causes for dandruff to grow due to stress, hormonal imbalance and medications and increased oil production in your body and much more.

If the scalp is mildly inflamed it could trigger dying skin cells grow. When the oils in the scalp is combined with the dead skin cells it can form a cluster of hair flakes. Then you can rid yourself of dandruff using apple cider vinegar, and get immediate relief.

Once you understand what causes dandruff you can treat it with greater efficiency. You can eliminate dandruff by using Apple cider vinegar. This apple cider vinegar can assist in replacing the pH balance of the scalp.

It can also add a shine your hair which shampoo is unable to provide. The most effective way to treat something is to repair and replenish what is missing , so it can find its balance. The body was created to self-heal itself.

For removing the dandruff using the apple cider vinegar first you must shampoo your hair using a mild shampoo. Do not fret about purchasing shampoo for dandruff because you'll never require it.

These shampoos can be costly and do not always fix the issue. The vinegar you apply can provide all the nutrients your scalp requires. After you've rinsed your hair, you're ready to apply to the solution of vinegar.

You'll need to mix an apple cider vinegar with warm water. It will take two portions of cider vinegar and one part of warm water.

If your dandruff has become difficult to treat and the combination isn't effective immediately You may want to test a stronger mix and include more vinegar, but less water. This is the best way to get rid of the dandruff by using Apple cider vinegar.

If you want to remove dandruff using Apple cider vinegar you can pour this vinegar along with warm water mix over the hair that has been rinsed and wet. It is also possible to put the mixture in the spray bottle and apply it to ensure that you're reaching all hair's areas.

The scent that comes from vinegar made of apples can be quite strong, so you might want to rinse it out , however it's not required unless you can't bear the smell.

The first outcomes shortly after you begin the treatment.

Chapter 8: The Yeast Infection

Anyone who has experienced an infection with yeast knows that they're not fun to suffer from. For us, the good news is that apple cider vinegar works as a potent natural remedy for relieving. If used properly it can aid in getting relief from the unpleasant symptoms.

If you're a female You may be suffering from burning or itching and redness, swelling and discomfort. If you're a man perhaps you are experiencing red dots, swelling dried skin or peeling, burning, or pain. If this is your case then apple cider vinegar is an excellent method to alleviate the symptoms.

In this section I will show you exactly how to use apple cider vinegar in order to relieve the yeast problem. If this remedy does not provide relief, then you could explore other home remedies that are available.

There are two different methods you can utilize apple cider vinegar to obtain relief from yeast infections. I'd like to talk about each of them with you today.

1. Bath and A.C.V.

One of the easiest methods to relieve the yeast infection is having bath. I know someone who has said that the bath was extremely beneficial to them and the addition of apple cider vinegar into the mixture will prove more beneficial.

All you need just add two cups apple cider vinegar into an icy bath, mix then lay down in the bath over 15 mins. After the bath, you can dry off, and then put on your underwear made of cotton It is recommended to wear a bathing suit.

2. A.C.V. Drink.

It's true that this is gross, but believe me when I tell you it certainly is. While it's not a good idea when you mix between 1 and two teaspoons apple cider vinegar in 8 ounces water and consume it, you will eventually feel that your symptoms be less severe. It is a popular treatment for a variety of ailments, such as acid reflux, as you are aware.

While it's not the best well-known remedy for yeast infections at home Apple cider vinegar could help you get rid of the symptoms. I would suggest bathing in it, since the flavor can be quite bad. If you're planning to attempt to pamper yourself internally, there's always yogurt. Yogurt is one of the most sought-after natural remedies you can find.

Chapter 9: Gout Pain

Apple cider vinegar is consumed externally and/or internally to reduce inflammation and pain associated with gout. In this section you'll find out how this type of vinegar can ease the symptoms of gout as well as how you can use it.

More than ever, gout becoming more prevalent around the world, who tend to treat their disease with medication. However, as the medications prescribed to treat gout have a variety of negative side effects, including some that are grave patients are looking for natural methods to manage their condition.

The benefits from Apple Cider Vinegar

There are numerous natural cures for gout however one of the most well-known ones can be found in the apple cider vinegar. Apple cider vinegar is used from the beginning as a home remedy for a wide variety of health problems that include Gout.

It must be pure Apple cider vinegar which isn't passedeurized or distillated. It might be difficult to locate in stores, but you can find this particular vinegar at health food stores and other specialty stores. You should be able observe a lot of sediment -- also known as by the name of the "mother"at the inside of the bottle.

The theory is that, when consumed as drink, this kind of cider alters the blood's pH which could aid in reducing high uric acid levels. When placed externally on the area of gout, it may aid in reducing swelling and ease discomfort.

How do I drink Apple Cider Vinegar to treat Gout

Blend 2 to 3 teaspoons vinegar into the water in a large glass. Take a glass of water every day, 2 or 3 times. Most people enjoy it this way, and the taste doesn't bother those who drink it. However, if you'd like to, you could add 2 teaspoons of honey to enhance the flavor.

How to Apply Apple Cider Vinegar Topically

The standard proportion for this application will be 1/2 (half) one cup of vinegar for 3 cups hot water. However, since you're going to submerge the joint into the solution,, you'll likely need to add more. Keep the ratio as it is.

For instance, to soak your feet, put in up to 2 to 12 cups hot water. It is important to check your water's temperature prior to immersing your feet or another area of the body where there is a gout.

Apple cider vinegar, raw and unfiltered is one of many natural remedies that you can avail to combat Gout. Other remedies that are popular include things like certain foods and veggies, herbs supplements, making certain adjustments on your eating habits modifications to your lifestyle, natural treatment, and more.

Chapter 10: A Natural Cleansing Agent

The apple cider vinegar can be a excellent natural cleaner. It serves so many functions that can be used in cooking and for use in the home that it is a must-have product in your home. You can also make huge savings in cash.

This natural cleaner is used to cleanse homes for over 10,000 years. It's also been utilized to improve the health of people and as a beauty boost for this length of time, too. Apple cider vinegar can be used to wash almost anything, both outside and inside.

An excellent solution for removing carpet staining. This can be used to remove food stains and pet staining. Add this to the dishwashing machine and observe how clean your dishes are. It can also remove hard water spots without difficulty. It can be added to your laundry and wash it to eliminate the stains that are there.

It can also brighten your clothing and stop their appearance from becoming dingy and faded. It helps in the setting of any dyes you may add and you could add it to the wash cycle so that you'll see your clothing cleaned more thoroughly.

A few people might be worried about the smell it might be leaving, but all you'll get is the scent of fresh, clean clothes There is no vinegar smell to be detected.

A difficult spot to clean is the oven with a grease stain and microwave too. Keep these areas clean and free of grime and grease. The removal of soap scum from showers, tiles and faucets can be an easy task thanks to the apple cider vinegar.

It can be used to remove dirt from countertops, floors as well as cabinets and even walls without worrying whether it will harm the areas or not. It is safe to use on almost any surface. There is no need for an additional disinfectant since apple cider vinegar can handle it also.

The applications for Apple cider vinegar can be numerous. You can try it on your trashcan or in your bathroom and in your kitchen. If you have troublesome pet areas, it can also work in those areas.

Doorknobs could be among the main sources of spreading germs. However, with just a quick wipe down using apple cider vinegar you will be able to remove any and all germs. Countertops as well as laundry rooms could benefit from this cost-effective cleaning product.

The apple cider vinegar can be an amazing general cleaner. It is a great cleaner for your windows, glass , and mirrors leaving a streak-free appearance and a shine you'll definitely love. It is simple to mix. Just simply add one-half cup apple cider vinegar and one-half cup of water, and you'll have a cleaner ready in a matter of minutes.

For tough stains for instance, in the bathroom for example, you can make use of apple cider vinegar at full strength. Use less of the cleaning agent as you can and then dry the area using the help of a paper towel. Be sure to not leave the cleaner on your floor, or it may cause damage to flooring.

There are so many ways to use the apple cider vinegar. If you're concerned about your environment or want to cut costs it is the best option for your home cleaning requirements.

Arthritis

Apple cider vinegar as a treatment for arthritis has been practiced for many years. There are numerous reasons behind this, which you must consider. Apple cider vinegar is actually a great source of numerous benefits for health and helping to ease arthritis pain is just one of them.

One thing you should know concerning arthritis is that the condition may be distinguished through the development of crystals of uric acids around joints. Apple cider vinegar is suggested to dissolve these crystals.

This is accomplished by malic acid, which makes up one the most active components in this kind of vinegar. The acid breaks the crystals into pieces so that they can be able to leave the body. It is important to remember that this doesn't stop the formation of crystals.

Inflammation is one of the things that people with arthritis suffer from too. This kind of vinegar could aid in this because it's an antioxidant in nature. The antioxidant properties will lessen the joint pain.

In addition, it is believed that this decrease will aid in slowing the progression of the disease. It is also a matter this vinegar may assist with. The acidic malic and acetic in the vinegar can also help your body fight infections.

How to Utilize Apple Cider Vinegar To Combat Arthritis Pain

There are two ways that people can use apple cider vinegar to treat arthritis. The other is via a compress. To make this happen you need to make a mixture that is one part apple cider vinegar and six portions water. Once the mixture gets hot, take it off the stove and soak a towel in it. Ring the excess out and place it on the joint pains.

Another method of administering the vinegar is to use it as an infusion. Most people drink one tablespoon twice per every day. It is possible to drink this vinegar on its own if don't mind the flavor. You can also add a tablespoon of vinegar to the water in a glass and drink it as is or make a tea using one teaspoon of honey that is natural.

There is no reason not to try apple cider vinegar to treat arthritis. The price of this natural cure is not too high while the rewards are numerous to count. Make sure to purchase a brand that is made of organic raw unfiltered apples for the greatest outcomes.

As A Thrush Treatment

The apple cider vinegar has become a well-known home treatment for thrush. Many people who have had enough of trying to get rid of their thrush using the traditional topical creams , pessaries and etc. are turning to natural remedies such as Apple cider vinegar.

Thrush (also known as yeast infections) can be described as an infection brought on by the growth the yeast-like fungus known as Candida Albicans. Most women are affected by vaginal thrush. This article will show you the methods to use apple cider vinegar to treat vaginal thrush.

It has been utilized to treat various illnesses for thousands of years. The minerals, trace elements, beneficial bacteria, enzymes and so on. which are found in the vinegar of raw apple cider is the reason for the healing qualities. Thrush isn't an exception.

However, you must make sure that the product is unpasteurized non-pasteurized, undistilled, and without preservatives or additives. It can be purchased from certain supermarkets or grocery stores however, your best option is to go to your local health food retailer. Here's how you can make use of this...

For a drink, mix the apple cider vinegar with two tablespoons into one glass of water. Drink it three times per every day. This can help manage this Candida Albicans fungi in your digestive tract.

For topical use, you can use it to wash your face. Simply add 2 tablespoons of vinegar in two four quarts of warm water, then gently wash with cotton pads. Repeat this process twice daily. Stop once the symptoms have gone away. The vinegar can help to balance the pH of your vagina (acidity) and helps to stop the growth of Candida fungi that live there.

Many women love bathing. To take a warm, gentle bath, add 2 glasses of vinegar from apple cider. Then remain in the tub for about 20 minutes or as long. It is important to open the vagina's mouth so that the warm liquid will penetrate the infection more effectively. If you want to repeat the procedure two times a day until symptoms of thrush go away.

The apple cider vinegar has become a loved home remedy for treating thrush. However, it's just one of many remedies at home for thrush that are available in the present. What women have observed is that certain remedies perform better than others, and what works for one person may not be effective for someone else.

There are also other issues to be considered. Some examples of factors that could help the Candida to grow include things like overuse of antibiotics and poor diet, steroids, weak immune system or weight issues, medication consumption, diabetes, etc. It is important to consider the above factors in order to get the best possible treatment to treat your thrush.

Treatment For Cellulite

Cellulite is the accumulation of fat below the skin's surface, around the buttocks, hips and the thighs. All races of women are affected by cellulite. It is most prevalent in overweight women, but doesn't exclusively affect slim women. Although cellulite isn't a sign of any illness however, it can be an issue for cosmetic reasons.

The skin is made up of band of elastic tissues which stretch from the skin to deep layers of muscle tissue. These bands are not elastic and when fat accumulates within the subcutaneous skin area there is only one method for it to move is to expand out onto the skin's surface. The connective tissue strands help to keep the skin from moving and give the appearance of dimples on the skin.

Cellulite formation is mostly due to an imbalance in the metabolism of fatty acids. Other factors such as inactivity and poor diet can also be at fault for the deposition of cellulite. Another reason for cellulite growth is the inadequate circulation of lymph and blood that causes build-up of toxins in the body.

There are a variety of remedies available for treating cellulite, and both natural solutions are preferred because of their security quality. ACV is among of the many natural remedies utilized to treat cellulite that has been used for more than two thousand years as weight loss therapy.

What is apple cider vinegar?

Pure Apple Cider Vinegar (ACV) is produced by crushing organically grown apples, and allow them to age within wooden barrels. This improves the natural fermentation process and lets the vinegar develop.

It is a powerful natural antibiotic that is made up of numerous essential minerals and trace elements like magnesium, calcium, potassium and phosphorous. It also contains chlorine as well as sulfur, sodium silicon, copper, iron and fluorine, which are essential for a healthy and healthy body.

The role of apple cider vinegar in treating cellulite

Apple cider vinegar is a great source of strength for immunity and helps treat numerous infections. It also boosts metabolism in the body and boosts thermogenesis.

Due to the increase in metabolic rate at the basal level, there is an increase in the burning of fat that is able to lower cholesterol levels and leads to weight loss.

Other micronutrients within apple cider vinegar such as lecithin and vitamin B6 also help in weight loss. Because weight loss is a key element of treatment for cellulite, apple cider vinegar is extremely beneficial.

The apple cider vinegar aids in removing the accumulation of fluids within the body, helping increase blood circulation.

* It's also believed to decrease appetite.

The apple cider vinegar is available in the form of capsules or liquid . The capsules are taken daily in two doses and could be increased to three doses per day in the event of need. The liquid form of the capsule can be consumed as two spoonfuls of an ice-cold glass to drink prior to every meal.

Athletes Foot

Apple cider vinegar is the most effective remedy to treat athlete's foot. It's the capability of this kind of vinegar to kill fungal infections that make it a great natural remedy for fungus that causes athlete's foot.

It is not only cheaper than prescription drugs and even over-the-counter medication, apple cider vinegar alleviates the itching caused by foot and ankle injuries, making it a gentleand natural solution to this painful and common issue. The best part is that you probably find it already in the pantry.

Athlete's Foot is a known, chronic ailment that is due to fungal growth that occurs on the feet. The infection is caused when the highly infectious tinea pedis fungus gets into the skin. The most commonly affected part on the feet is the area between toes which is particularly humid and warm. However it could also affect the rest part of your foot.

If the fungus of athlete's foot is given the chance to grow, it can begin with an itchy , red rash generally starting between the fifth and fourth toe. If the infection isn't treated, the skin can be extremely soft and sensitive to sensation.

In the cases of the most severe those edges around the affected area may become white, and the skin may fall off, creating an oily discharge.

To stop this debilitating condition to combat this ailment, many have repeatedly turned to cider vinegar made from apples. This kind of vinegar is made of the liquid taken from the crushed apples. It is made with yeast and sugar to stimulate fermentation, and convert the sugars into alcohol.

It's in the second fermentation stage that bacteria that produce acetic acid convert the alcohol to vinegar.

This product is acidic and is a treatment for feet that are raw broken, cracked, or damaged by the fungus which causes athlete's foot. It not only relieves the itchiness that persists due to the condition but but it is also believed to cleanse the body of the fungal infection that causes the condition. It might not have the best scent but the relief felt after feet with sore feet touch the vinegar will be worth it.

A foot soak is a great solution to combat foot fungus, also known as athlete's foot. Simply mix one portion of all-natural apple cider vinegar and one part warm water, and let it let it soak for around 20 minutes. The feet should be washed by using a mild soap prior to and following the treatment.

It is important to ensure that your feet are completely dry after the treatment to avoid it from spreading to the humid environment. If needed, it's possible to do this kind of treatment two times per day. In accordance with how severe the issue feet must be cleared of the fungus within a period of one to two weeks of routine treatment at home.

In less severe cases of athlete's femur Utilize a washcloth, or a cotton ball that has been soaked with apple cider vinegar. The cloth should be gently rubbed on the affected areas. This method is particularly effective for children who might not be able to sit for a bath, due to the fact that the combination of vinegar and the rub of the washcloth will instantly relieve the itching that is caused by fungus.

It is recommended to take basic precautions to reduce your risk of contracting the fungus because preventing the fungus can be much more straightforward than treating the latter is a lot more difficult. The most crucial step to take is to keep your feet dry, particularly between your toes.

Check that the atmosphere inside your socks is not conducive for fungal growth. Socks made of wool, cotton and other organic materials permit feet to breathe while remaining dry.

If you find that your feet often sweat make sure your socks are dry and clean regardless of changing your socks in the middle of the daytime. Select shoes that are well ventilated, and give them time to dry before you wear them again.

It is also essential to limit the risk for exposure to the sun by using water-resistant sandals or shoes when you go to locker rooms, showers in public and any other moist and warm place which could harbor tinea pedis. By taking treatment of feet, and cleaning them regularly with natural apple cider vinegar can ensure that the foot fungus is eliminated and doesn't get back.

Fibroids

There's a lot of talk about fibroids as well as Apple cider vinegar (ACV) and how it helps shrink fibroids naturally. ACV is among the most frequently recommended natural treatments for a wide range of ailments and conditions.

One reason it is a well-known natural cure is that it is readily used in many kitchens it is fairly inexpensive and has little or negative side negative effects. While there isn't any scientific evidence to back the numerous health benefits of the use of ACV however, it remains an extremely popular natural cure.

ACV is a natural remedy. many people have praised the advantages of ACV for a myriad of illnesses, including diabetes weight loss and heartburn, psoriasis, dry scalp, dry skin constipation, dry hair, high cholesterol the ear and nail fungus Dandruff, arthritis kidney stones, warts yeast infections, jock itch etc.

Although there is any scientific evidence that ACV could be effective for all of these conditions however, there are plenty of positive reviews from those who have tried ACV to treat any variety of illnesses.

The most important thing to consider about research in the field of science with regards to many home remedies, is the fact that there isn't any incentive for huge sums of money to be spent research on remedies like ACV because it is unlikely to be feasible to patent ACV because it is widely accessible.

The Fibroids as well as Apple Cider Vinegar

The acidity of ACV could be the reason for its ability to fight off many illnesses and is the reason it is regarded as antifungal, antibacterial and antiviral. It is also a source of various minerals and vitamins that our bodies require in addition to enzymes as well as essential anti-inflammatory properties that can all assist in fighting off various ailments.

A lot of Eastern experts believe illness and diseases such as fibroids, are result of an acidic condition within the body. Helping the body to become more alkaline will help combat various ailments and ailments and build an overall healthier body.

It is important to remember that even though its acidic properties are a reason why ACV is often cited for its beneficial properties it has when applied topically, when consumed in the internal system, ACV does have an actual alkaline effect on the body, helping to elevate the pH from one that is acidic to an alkaline level that can aid the body to improve its health.

Toxins in our bodies could also increase the chance of developing various ailments and conditions, including the growth of tumors called fibroids. Another advantage of ACV is its ability in detoxifying the body.

Being overweight is yet another risk factor in the development of fibroid ACV may aid in weight loss that indirectly aids to combat a myriad of health conditions and diseases that are a result of weight such as fibroids.

These health benefits and others that are associated with ACV is why women who suffer from fibroids frequently boast about the ability of ACV to reduce fibroids naturally in the absence of any scientific evidence.

How do you use apple cider vinegar to help with fibroids

There's no set amount however, many women drink 1 tablespoon or 2 teaspoons of ACV each day. Since drinking pure ACV (undiluted) can chip away the tooth enamel and result in burns on the delicate areas of the mouth and throat it is recommended to mix it into an liquid.

ACV is usually mixed ACV with 8 ounces of water tea , or milk (soy almond milk, etc., are superior to dairy milk particularly for people with fibroids).

Another way to protect yourself from ACV should be to keep clear from ACV supplements as studies have demonstrated that these supplements could permanently harm the tissues in the esophagus.

Best apple cider vinegar for fibroids

The first suggestion is to utilize ACV instead of other kinds of vinegar (e.g. white vinegar) since ACV is made of apples. This is why it has the highest amount of minerals, vitamins, and trace minerals our bodies require to stay healthy.

Other varieties of vinegar, like white vinegar don't have the same properties.

Another important thing to consider is various methods utilized to produce ACV several of which reduce the positive characteristics of ACV. This is the reason why the majority of the products that are sold in stores be avoided for use in the home since they lack beneficial properties.

The most beneficial apple cider vinegar you can make an alternative to conventional remedies is one made from organic apples. It is unfiltered, raw and fermented in traditional ways (unpasteurized). It is important to mention that it is a "mother" which is the place where most of the beneficial properties from apple cider vinegar can be found.

Type 2 Diabetes

It has been utilized for a long time by people from all walks of life and has a wide range of advantages. Let's take a look at three benefits that you need to be aware of...

1. Blood Sugar Control. One of the main benefits you will reap by using the apple cider vinegar recipe is the stabilization of the blood sugar level. For those who suffer from Type 2

diabetes, this is an advantage you'll be looking to note down.

Mixing a tablespoon of apple cider vinegar with one cup of water is a fantastic method to reduce the blood sugar spike you might experience after eating an adipose-rich meal.

2. pH Balancer. Apple cider vinegar can be an effective way to maintain your pH levels and ensure that they're within an acceptable range.

If you're one who consumes a large quantity of meat in your daily plan, you're more acidic than generally considered healthy.

A diet high in protein does produce this effect and if you're not trying to incorporate a broad range of vegetables and fresh fruits in your daily diet there is a chance that you are in for some unpleasant negative side negative effects.

This could include thoughts that...

Fatigue,

Dizziness,

Inability to concentrate and also

Rapid heart rate or fluctuations of blood pressure.

Despite the fact that it's acidic however, apple cider vinegar will be more alkaline when it is in your system. This means it will help in removing you from the extremely acidic state which can make you healthier in general.

3. Allergy Control. Apple cider vinegar could help in fighting allergies that are seasonal. It could help in removing the sinus mucus which makes breathing easier.

If you're one who relies heavily on allergy medications that are available over the counter You may be aware that these frequently have the potential for causing individuals to feel extremely sleepy. Consider a natural remedy that you can use, and you might be able to avoid this.

As you can see, there are a myriad of reasons to incorporate apple cider vinegar into your diet routine These reasons are only the beginning of the Iceberg. There are a myriad of other fantastic ways to use cider vinegar made from apple, therefore make sure to do some study and ensure you're not omitting any of the benefits that come from this potent ingredient.

Although managing the disease isn't easy, Type 2 diabetes is not something you have to simply endure. There are simple adjustments you can make to your routine that will decrease your weight as well as your level of blood sugar. Be patient for a while, the longer you stick with it the easier it becomes.

Heartburn

The apple cider vinegar can be a traditional remedy to eliminate heartburn. In fact, it's the TOP alternative to treat acid reflux and heartburn.

Recipe for Relief

The use of apple cider vinegar to treat heartburn relief is very easy. Simply mix two Tablespoons of vinegar made from apple in 1/2 cup of apple juice or water. Drink it right after every meal. If you are suffering from acid reflux after having a the most hefty meal, you should increase the quantity in apple cider vinegar, and reduce the quantity of juice or water.

Another option is mixing the following ingredients into a "cocktail" consisting of these:

* 1 quart apple juice

* 1 pint purple grape juice

* 1/2 cup apple cider vinegar

Drink 1/2 cup after every meal for heartburn relief.

Recipes using apple cider vinegar to get rid of heartburn are diverse. The reason for this is that the bodies of each person also differ in a variety of ways. You can experiment with various amounts of vinegar made from apple cider until you discover the one that works best for you.

Certain people have discovered that one or the other brand performs better for them. The reason for this is due to variations in the physical makeup.

What Apple Cider Vinegar helps Heartburn

A little research has been conducted regarding the efficacy in the use of vinegar made from apple to provide heartburn relief. Therefore, it's difficult to determine how apple cider vinegar relieves heartburn.

It is believed that the acid content of vinegar is a signal to your stomach that it is not producing acid. Perhaps, in this way the apple cider vinegar works similar to prescription drugs used to "shut down" the stomach's acid pump to prevent heartburn.

Apple cider vinegar doesn't taste great to the majority of people. Due to this, people have tried eating a handful of slices of apple following meals and have been rid of heartburn this way. Some apples are not effective to relieve heartburn, however. Certain people prefer the green variety, such as Granny Smith.

Others suggest Jonagold apples to ease heartburn. A few people recommend eating a couple of slices of Jonagold apple along with some spears of dill pickle. This vinegar is apple cider for heartburn, without resorting to simple vinegar.

Bacterial Vagiosis

BV, also known as bacterial vagiosis isn't a pleasant disease. It can cause the outside and inside of the vagina to become swollen and itchy. It may also cause the discharge of unpleasant smells emanating from your vagina.

In addition, you could be experiencing constipation, cramps or bleeding due to your BV. It can be a real cause of miserable and end your sexual pleasure. This is a condition which women are usually eager to treat.

Eliminating Bacteria

The conventional method to treat BV that is known as a bacterial ailment, is to eliminate the bacteria responsible for the infection. The doctor may recommend that you take antibiotics.

But, antibiotics destroy all bacteria, and the issue that women often don't realize is that a woman's vagina is supposed to be a reservoir of healthy bacteria that protect it from infection.

The Balance is Changing:

The reason why apple cider vinegar functions extremely well in treating BV is because it is mildly acidic. It has the ability change the pH in the vagina in a way that will let good bacteria stay healthy and prevent bad bacteria from forming.

You can also alter the vaginal environment instead of completely eliminating all the bacteria using antibiotics.

A Vinegar Bath:

If you're looking to make use of apple cider vinegar in order to alleviate symptoms of BV, one simple method to achieve this is to have an apple cider vinegar soak. Begin by taking in a warm, shallow, and shallow bath. Mix in around half to a full cup of the vinegar to your bathing water. Be cautious not to use too much vinegar as it could trigger an intense burning sensation as you relax in the bath tub.

A bath with apple cider vinegar can be beneficial however you shouldn't be doing frequently. Be aware that you're trying to restore the balance of your vagina. If you are tipping the scales too much in the opposite direction could be a cause for your problem to become worse.

A Vinegar Douche:

As with a bath in vinegar, a vinegar-based douche ought to be thoroughly dilute. One one teaspoon apple cider vinegar mixed with the form of two cups of water will be sufficient. In addition, like the vinegar bath, don't wash too often. Every day, once is enough to complete the task.

Drinking Vinegar:

Drinking a glass of apple cider vinegar can be an effective way to avoid BV but it might not be as beneficial like a bath or a douche to treat an current BV outbreak.

However using apple cider vinegar to get relief from BV, particularly in the event that you are planning to consume it must be handled with caution. Because it's slightly acidic, it isn't necessary or desire excessive amounts of it within your system. Therefore, take it with care and you'll see that it will provide you with important relief from BV.

Chapter 11: The History Of Apple Cider

Vinegar was probably a fortunate error, made in various parts of the globe. A bottle of beer or wine was discovered too long and a legend of food was created. The history of Vinegar goes back at least 8000 yearsago; vessels with vinegar-related traces that date back to 6000 B.C.E were discovered within Egypt in Egypt and China.

We've reported that approximately 5,000 B.C.E. that the Babylonians used vinegar made of dates for a calming and condiment. They also started to explore aromatic varieties of vinegar made with spices and herbs. The use to use vinegar for cooking was known for a long time and the first doctor to prescribe vinegar for a variety of ailments and health issues included Hippocrates (around around 400 B.C.E.).

Hippocrates was long known to utilize apple cider vinegar as a remedy for health. Since then, many home remedy books and the stories of older women have all advised the use of this vinegar. The doctor Dr. Jarvis wrote a book in the year 1958, describing the advantages of apple cider to the health. According to his advice cider vinegar must be mixed with honey sweet and a teaspoon of it is recommended to be consumed every day. In the 1970s, the popularity of vinegar made from apple cider had been increasing once more. After reading the book, his proponents came up with the apple cider vinegar diet plan to lose weight.

A vase with traces that date back to the time of the Pharaoh were found in Egypt which suggests the fact that Egyptians knew about the use of vinegar and made use of to preserve food, like the people of Babylonian and Persian used to do. Vinegar was used to transport food items on long distances. Mixing together with water and saline, the farmers, and travelers utilized it in earlier times to quench thirst.

Vinegar to treat disease and other health issues has been utilized since Hippocrates (around around 460-377 B.Sc.). The Greek physician, known by the name of"the "father of medicine"" utilized vinegar to cleanse injuries as well as treat lacerations that were open and infected and advised a vinegar and honey combination to treat respiratory problems that persist.

"Mother" in Apple Cider Vinegar "Mother" is in Apple Cider Vinegar

It is believed that Apple Cider Vinegar includes an powerful "mother," the sediment-like and cobweb-like material that is visible even in nonfiltered ACV products. The mother is a concentrated source of enzymes and bacteria that are what make ACV famous for its anti-fungal, antiviral and antibacterial healing properties. While some may be dissuaded from the ACV bottles due to their water content, the element is the result of a special process that keeps apple's nutrients as well as enzymes during the fermentation process , and provides specific curative properties for the ACV.

The history of Babylonians from the Babylonians to Samurai warriors

Vinegar is among the oldest methods of fermentation known to the human race dating back from Babylonians to warriors of the samurai. The first fermentation process is through wine, which is where vinegar was first produced. The Babylonians date back to 5000 BC were the first to make date palm wine and the Egyptians created their barley wines. In the 2500 BC period The Aryans created an apple wine that was soured which was the precursor to apple ciders, originating from an old nomadic group. The term 'cider' originates of the Phoenician' Shekar,' which is a strong drink or wine. This is how the Babylonians and the Aryans as well as they, the Phoenicians, Greeks, and Romans came the soiled Apple wine recipe.

Then the people started developing Apple Cidre vinegar as a result of their soiled apple wine (Rose 2006).

The vinegar of apple cider has been utilized in medical treatments for hundreds of centuries... It is commonly utilized to treat a range of ailments, such as poisoning by mushrooms and dandruff. It also helps with tooth pain. In during the US Civil War and World War I It was utilized to treat wounds from battle. Japanese soldiers of the Samurai were instructed to drink it to boost their strength and strength. The ancient Persians took a dilution of vinegar and apple cider to prevent the formation of fatty tissues within the body. Romans utilized the fire and vinegar during their Alpine conquer to break rock. Vinegar has been utilized to preserve food items for many years and is an effective cleaning agent today. In short, the records of history show an apple cider vinegar that is found all over the globe is utilized in numerous ways (Rose 2006).

Ancient Greece

The ancient Greece Oxycrat is the main commonly consumed drink consumed in the early years of Greece the drink of the people. Mixing vinegar, water and sugar were stored in individual vase (oxides). A remarkable doctor,

Hippocrates, whose doctrines were the basis of Western civilization up to in the 1800s, i.e. during more than 2,000 years. advised him on how to treat sores, wounds and breath-related diseases.

The Romans

The Romans were known to drink "posca," a combination of vinegar and water. It is available for sale on the streets in the present, similar to coconut sellers. Posca was thought to provide energy and you could also get drunk by drinking wine. (Fortem Posca, Vinum erbium facit). The praetorian offered an ointment-soaked sponge to Jesus at the altar.

It was not a sign of cruelty however it was a symbol for the soldier's burial to a man who was on the cross. Acetabulum, which was a glass bowl with half vinegar and a table that was accompanied by people who would drink small portions of bread with their meals to aid digestion. It was often present at Roman banquets.

Vinegar was the main ingredient in recipes made by Apicius who was a well-known Epicurean chef during Roman times. The current version, Columella, has left some vinegar recipes. acid yeast is utilized to aid in fermentation, and incandescent bars along with hot fir cones were put in wine to cleanse their properties.

The Romans were known to have a variety of vinegar sauces, from the simplest to the popular garum, the bizarre combination of various ingredients blended with vinegar. Vinegar also served to make an "acetarie" food item, vegetables, meat salads and other vegetables that were served with the main meals. The Romans developed the technique of marinating fish that was fried. Then, in His Naturalism History, Pliny the Elder suggests vinegar for treating various ailments and to improve the quality of life.

Vinegar was always readily available to Roman legionaries. Their breakfast before fight was which was a salad consisting from onions, garlic and rue, goat's milk, and coriander coated with vinegar and oil.

In the course of military operations, vinegar was also utilized to quench thirst. It was combined with water to cleanse the skin to prevent and treat wounds caused by camp life as well as minor injuries.

Hannibal Barca, the famous general of the Carthaginian army (247-183 B.C.) was a famous general who crossed the Alps with knights, foot soldiers, and elephants in the Piccolo San Bernardo Pass and therefore avoided the Roman-dominated ocean during the crucial battle that fought between Rome as well as Carthage. It's a cult occasion. It's not evident why he went over the Alps. The roads are narrow and twisting, making it difficult for elephants of enormous size. Hannibal had enormous branches in between the rocks that blocked the path and set the rocks on burning. After he put vinegar on hot stones. The stone was brittle, and soldiers would smash them to pass through the animals and soldiers.

In The Middle Ages And Beyond

Middle age

The method of making vinegar developed in the Middle Ages, and Agresto was initially made with green grapes which were able to counterbalance the flavoring fat, thanks to their fresh and light acidity.

In 1394, the newly formed vinegar producers' association of Orleans placed the secrecy of manufacturing technology at risk of being ejected from its unit. This is why Orleans vinegar is widely used and business is flourishing. In 1580, the town as well as its surrounding areas included 33 mills for vinegar as local wine that was not particularly acidic and fruity, it was ideal to make vinegar.

The geographical position of Orleans was advantageous: It was also the last port on the maritime route for products coming from west. Ships traveling on the river were extremely slow due to the water shortage, and by the time wine arrived at the port it was ready to be processed into vinegar through the correct mixing with the local wine.

Vinegar , the plague

The Black Death spread all over Europe and affected one of three people during the early 14th century. The outbreak of the disease was observed each year by different levels.

It is thought that vinegar can be excellent in preventing disease, and the inhabitants from Marseilles protected themselves from "fever-creating" atmospheric conditions in 1720 which was the year of the final major outbreak in the west of Europe. They kept a sponge swept with vinegar "under your nose" but never breathing through their mouths as well as swallowing saliva. Nurses aided doctors with the vinegar basin where the physicians could cleanse their hands prior to patients were able to feel the pain. Once the plague had slowed down. they could clean the insides of homes that housed patients were sick were washed by using vinegar.

Vinegar from the four thieves.

A bandage treated with vinegar was put on the forehead of Monatti, one of the body's carriers to prevent infections, according to Manzoni. There were four of them (some people claim seven) could wash the town of scot-free during the outbreak of plague in 1720 in Marseille due to the ablutions and vinegar gargles, whose ingredients are not known.

They were eventually executed for robbery and sackcloth, however, the lives of these four were saved thanks to the vinegar they left behind known as"the Vinegar from the Four Thieves. The four-year-old's vinegar Robberies was formulated by an French expert, Misette Godard, based on the original Marseilles recipe, which included various spice, cloves and camphor and wormwood. It also contained 3 pints vinegar.

Vinegar and Cholera

An infected disease that was once prevalent in distant regions in Asia. It's still prevalent across several countries of Europe and is frequently confused with acute gastroenteritis and it shares many resemblances. Cholera was treated with vinegar at any time in the past. In the government of Vienna issued an act in the latter century (1830 and 1884) due to the outbreak of cholera, which required people were required to clean your hands in vinegar prior and after visiting along with fruits and vegetables prior to eating. Cholera is spread through water, which is why preventative actions and disinfection of food are well-known.

Recent research conducted by Franco Mecca (Franco Angeli Editore) ("Wine vinegar generally, to help prevent outbreaks of cholera and other cholera-related outbreaks") suggests that vinegar is the ability to have a "simple and noticeable" disinfectant impact on cholera as well as various intestinal pathogens. Within 30 seconds to 1-2 minutes, the vibrios found on the surface of fruits and vegetables that come in contact with vinegar will be destroyed.

Vinegar is a product for beauty

The royals and princes of the world made use of vinegar in the past century as a cosmetic. The King of Portugal and Queen of Holland and the queen of Belgium and the princess of Wales were chosen, according to the advertisement within "Il Secolo" the 15th of February in 1873.

It was used to declare "that provides water with a pleasant smell and also has tone and soothing qualities." stops chilblains developing and also strengthens the muscles. These ads also include ammonia vinegar, which was used as a disinfectant for hospitals, lazar homes and "other areas where breathing problems could occur." Vinegar also was used to clean both in the past and present. As Misette Godard has pointed out that the current situation in European cities of the time is best assessed by comparing it to the present day Calcutta.

Vinegar, a multi-purpose product

Vinegar is a multi-functional drug. Women smelt vinegar during the 19th century in order to revive their senses, in the event that their corset was too tight or for headaches. The housekeeper would leave an open bottle of vinegar near a person suffering from flu to help prevent illness from those who came to visit him/her.

Our ancestors utilized vinegar for the production of syrups, emulsions and salts, decoctionsand mouthwash sublimates, lotions soap for the eyes, eyewash, and buffers. Vinegar is also utilized for massaging, rinsing football, gargling, shaving, fomenting inhaling, showering plastering, bandaging, and many other purposes.

The waves of immigration from Germany and Eastern Europe over the years led to a love affair with beer, and it also cleared in the Midwest-- a region much more welcoming to growing grains and leaps than the Atlantic shoreline. In recognition of its origins Ciders are starting to return to bars across the country which makes this robust beverage an important surviving drink.

Apple cider vinegar for Blood Sugar and diabetes

A glass of apple cider vinegar often considered to be a natural method to regulate blood sugar levels especially for those who suffer from insulin resistance.

If taken prior to eating the consumption of a high-carb meal vinegar can slow down the rate of stomach draining and prevents blood sugar spikes.

It also increases insulin levels of sensitivity. This helps your body in moving more sugar out of your blood stream and in your body cells the blood glucose levels are reduced.

Apple cider vinegar is a source of internet links to a range of wellness benefits including weight loss, as well as reducing cold symptoms. Can it help people who suffer from diabetes mellitus?

Researchers haven't yet been able to confirm all of the claims of wellness regarding apple cider vinegar through extensive research studies. There is evidence to suggest the apple cider vinegar could offer specific benefits in the treatment of diabetes mellitus.

Diabetic problems are a constant problem that results in a inability to manage blood glucose levels appropriately. As per The Globe Wellness Company (THAT) in 1980, about 100 million people had diabetes mellitus. The incidence has dramatically increased in the past couple of years and reached around 422 million as of 2014.

Amazingly, only a small percent of vinegar made from apple cider is needed for these outcomes.

According to studies that apple cider vinegar may have the potential to impact different kinds of diabetes by a variety of ways.

Certain research studies like this study from 2018, has the connection with apple cider vinegar as well as lower blood sugar levels.

Many people believe the apple cider vinegar may be beneficial for people with diabetes mellitus who need to control their blood sugar levels.

There are two major types of diabetes-related issues: type 1 . And type 2. In type 1 the pancreatic gland is unable to produce insulin because the body's immune system attacks the cells that create insulin. Anyone suffering from type 1 diabetes will need to supplement their insulin intake.

The body's cells are able to be less prone to the effects of glucose reduction insulin, type 2 occurs. This means that the body absorbs significantly less sugar, leaving lots of glucose flowing through the bloodstream.

The diet plan can have a positive impact on the type 2 diabetes mellitus. It is an important aspect to take into account for those with type one.

Although apple cider vinegar is an effective and low-risk addition to a diabetic-friendly diet, the research studies on the vinegar are nascent and have reached a common conclusion about the effects it has on blood sugar levels.

Study

The research on the impact of apple cider vinegar on blood glucose levels often aren't and also have mixed outcomes.

A majority of research studies that have examined the vinegar apple cider have examined its potential to lower blood sugar levels. A study conducted in 2018 examined both its long- and short-term results and found that a majority of the results favored the teams using vinegar, though not usually with a significant amount. Teams were plagued by both types of diabetes-related issues.

The research suggests Apple cider vinegar caused the slightest, most significant reduction in HbA1c results after 8-12 weeks. The HbA1c levels reflect the levels of blood sugar in an individual throughout a period of time, whether weeks or even months.

On a brief basis, groups taking apple cider vinegar experienced a substantial increase in blood sugar levels 30 minutes after having eaten the vinegar. The differences between vinegar and control teams diminished after this timeframe.

Other studies have attempted to discover the mechanism that cause this drop in blood sugar levels. A study that was randomized, cross-sectional and randomized in 2015 suggested the apple cider vinegar may improve the way the body absorbs blood glucose. It could also improve the level of insulin sensitivity within the muscle mass of skeletal.

Apple cider vinegar is composed of acetic acid. It certain scientists claim takes on less weight. The source of the vinegar like apple cider, influences its impact to the human body.

One study conducted in 2017 on computer mice showed that computer mice who received vinegar dosages saw a decrease in body weight, and fat circulation.

Problems with weight can lead to the progression of type 2 diabetes mellitus.

Although this study doesn't indicate that the exact results will occur in humans however, it does point out the mechanisms that could cause a reduction in blood sugar levels after taking apples cider vinegar.

Apple cider vinegar's effects on people with type 1 diabetes are the subject of less definite research. The last study to examine this was in the year 2010 and discovered that 2 tbsps (tbs) in vinegar may help reduce hyperglycemia or high sugar levels following meals.

A different research study from 2007however suggested the use of apple cider vinegar, which might cause symptoms to get more severe. It could hinder the process of clearing the stomach is cleared, and can influence the administration of sugar in people who frequently use insulin.

The characteristics of research studies and the lack of research studies on apple cider vinegar and type 1 diabetes make it difficult for doctors to suggest apple cider vinegar as a suitable treatment for people suffering from this type of diabetes mellitus.

Consuming apple cider vinegar isn't likely to cause major damage. Always monitor degrees to see if it is functioning and make nutritional adjustments according to the guidelines.

4 teaspoons (20 milliliters) from apple cider vinegar prior to eating has been found to significantly lower blood sugar levels following consumption.

It should be mixed with a few 8 ounces of water. It can also be eaten prior to eating the preparation of a high-carb meal.

If taken prior to an a dish that is high in fiber or low in carbs, Apple cider vinegar does not significantly lower blood sugar levels.

Drinking 4 tsps (20 milliliters) from apple cider vinegar that has been thinned in water prior to eating a dish with high carbs will help reduce blood glucose spikes.

What exactly is the best way to use Apple Cider Vinegar For Diabetes

1. Apple Cider Vinegar And Water

What You Do You

2 tablespoons of ACV

2 Tbsps of water

- 1 oz cheese

What To Do?

Mix the ACV and drink it as the water. Drink the mix, along with your favorite celebrity, prior to getting to the bed.

How often do you need to Do This

Do it for one week, as well with consulting your physician after the results. Follow their advice.

What is the reason? This Why It Works

ACV contains acetic acid which is recognized as having antiglycemic effects. Additionally, vinegar and cheese might have a collaborative influence.

2. Cinnamon And Apple Cider Vinegar

What You Are Looking For

1 tsp ACV

3/4 tsp ground cinnamon

1 tsp of Stevia

What To Do?

Mix all active ingredients and mix the ingredients in recipe from this blog post.

How often do you need to Do This

2 times per every day. Talk to a medical professional results of the article.

The Reasons This How It Works

Cinnamon may help lower blood sugars in the bloodstream during fasting (4). Although the drink is sweetened with stevia but it has an glycemic score of none and isn't taken up by digestive tracts.

3. Honey And Apple Cider Vinegar

What You Are Looking For

1 tsp ACV

1 teaspoon of honey (and maybe less).

1/2 cup of water.

What to Do.

Mix all the ingredients together and drink recipe dishes.

What is the best way to Perform This.

Two or three times per every day. Consult your doctor about the results.

The Reasons This How It Works.

Honey is a great alternative to the acidic taste of ACV. It might not have the same effect on blood sugar levels as sugar does, but it could be a balanced, healthy substitute.

Care.

If you have diabetes mellitus that is controlled, try honey for a short period of time. If not, it's much better to avoid the use of honey or replace it by using the use of stevia.

4. Sodium Bicarbonate And Apple Cider Vinegar.

What Do You Need.

2 tablespoons of ACV.

1/2 teaspoon in cooking soft drinks.

A variety of orange wedges.

What to Do.

Include a quarter tsp of cooking soft drinks to the stem of a glass.

Place the entire ACV directly into the stemless glass, as well as mixing thoroughly.

Drink the alcohol blend.

It is possible to draw, or drink those orange slices. This will eliminate the bitter taste of ACV in your mouth.

How often should you Do This.

Three times per day.

Care.

If you're experiencing digestive issue that affects the mouthor esophagus stomach, or digestive tracts, consult your doctor before using this treatment.

Anyone who wants to take apple cider vinegar must be able to reduce 1- 2 tablespoons of vinegar made from apple using the form of a large glass.

Consume it before eating or before getting ready for bed, as it has the greatest potential to minimize impact on blood glucose.

Like the majority of of vinegar, a person must avoid eating the vinegar that is not mixed with apple cider. In its own it can cause discomfort in the stomach or even damage enamel on the teeth.

Apple cider vinegar can also be an adaptable food preparation ingredient. People can use it in soup dressings, salad dressings sauces, dressings, as well as in sauces, as in combination with many kinds of meats and fish.

The public is likely to see the ranges of apple cider vinegar on sale. This kind of vinegar made from apple cider is crystal clear and does not have any shade.

For POLYCYSTIC OVARIAN SYNDROME (PCOS)

What exactly is PCOS?

The state of mind that fluctuatesa term commonly used for females, is a symptom caused by hormonal fluctuations. One of the endocrine issues are PCOS i.e. polycystic ovarian disorders in which the female's hormones are not functioning properly. The polycystic disorder of ovarian cysts (PCOS) is an hormonal issue that is associated with irregular menstrual cycles, high levels of androgen hormones as well as ovarian cysts. It can also be a sign of insulin resistance.

To study the effect of vinegar on hormones and metabolic indicators and also the ovulatory aspect of PCOS Seven people searching for non-pharmacological treatments for PCOS were given a drink containing 15 grams of apple cider vinegar each day for 90-110 days. The research suggests vinegar's potential to enhance ovulatory function by raising the insulin sensitivity in PCOS clients, thereby hindering the need for medical therapy. The consumption of vinegar could reduce cost for clinical treatment and the time required for treatment for anovulation, insulin resistance and inability to conceive for those who suffer from PCOS.

Three-month research studies revealed that women suffering from PCOS who consumed alcohol 1 tablespoon (15 mg) in apple cider vinegar, containing 100ml or about 7 ounces of liquid after dinner had increased hormone levels and observed longer durations of normalization.

Further research studies are needed to verify these findings 1 teaspoon (15 mg) each day is to be a good dose for improving PCOS symptoms and signs.

In a typical day, drinking one tablespoon (15 milliliters) in apple cider vinegar along with 100ml or around 7 ounces of water following eating dinner could increase the symptoms and signs of PCOS.

What is the trigger for PCOS?

In a normal, healthy and balanced woman's body, both female hormones for sex and small male sex hormonal agents (androgen) are created to help the normal advancement of the ovary every menstrual. When you suffer from PCOS the body experiences an inequities between these hormones i.e. the ovaries start spinning out more androgen and causing irregular menstrual cycles as well as facial hair growth loss of hair, fertility issues as well as the condition known as hirsutism.

Typically, during each menstrual cycle, many eggs are released (a process called the ovulation). In this type of endocrine disorder, eggs in the cavities that are thought of as roots inside the ovaries don't get developed and are not released from the ovaries , forming tiny cysts within the Ovaries i.e. polycystic Ovaries.

Polycystic Ovarian Disorder (PCOS) is among the most common endocrine disorders in women, which affects the body in many ways. PCOS is, in fact is among the main causes of inability of women to conceive who are in their reproductive years. Females who suffer PCOS,

PCOS their ovaries produce more androgens than female hormones that regulate reproduction.

The treatment of PCOS is usually complex as there is no cause or result-related connection. Most often, drugs and lifestyle adjustments are recommended for treating PCOS. There are specific home treatments that can help in dealing with PCOS.

How do you utilize apple cider vinegar to treat PCOS

It's easy and takes almost no effort. To combat PCOS consume 1 up to 2 tablespoons in apple cider vinegar each day. You do not need to drink the vinegar raw. Instead you can use it to dress your salad or mix 2 spoons the vinegar with water , and take it in.

What are the benefits of using apple cider vinegar.

In this particular test 7 women with PCOS consumed one tablespoon in apple cider vinegar every day. In addition apple cider vinegar also helps in weight loss, which is an added benefit for females suffering from PCOS.

Benefits from Apple Cider Vinegar for Women who suffer from PCOS.

The resistance to insulin can be a common characteristic of females with PCOS and is also associated to having difficulty with ovulating. Insulin sensitizing drugs such as Metformin and Metformin, are used to combat Anovulation, as well as irregular periods in women with PCOS to increase fertility.

Vinegar is made up of acetic acids as in tiny amounts of amino acid, vitamin comprised of vitamin C and mineral salts. It is believed to offer many benefits like being antibacterial as well as aiding in dealing with infections, offering cardiovascular security, as well as maintaining food intake.

A 2013 study looked at the effect from vinegar's effects on the ovulation cycle levels as and the levels of hormones for females suffering from PCOS. 7 women aged between 21-40 years of age consumed 100ml of a drink comprising 15 grams in apple cider vinegar referred to as apple vinegar by study daily for 90 to 110 days. 2 of the women were overweight, and one was obese.

In the course of 40 days drinking alcohol apple cider vinegar, four of 7 people were ovulating and began with regular durations, which included of females who were considered to be overweight. Two of the remaining individuals had ovulated in greater forty days. One lady, described as being sterile for two years, continued to drink the vinegar made from apple cider for a further 2 months , in addition to the study's 90-day period and was also thought to be the idea of.

The researchers concluded that vinegar increased the resistance to insulin and also the Ovulatory activity in people in similar manner to Metformin and could also be effective for non-obese as overweight females suffering from PCOS who are insulin-resistant. Further research is needed to determine the effectiveness of vinegar in females who suffer from PCOS for non-pharmacological treatment.

Apple CIDER VINEGAR TO HELP WEIGHT LOSS

Vinegar can help people lose weight by enhancing the sensation of weight loss and decreasing the amount of food consumed in the day.

In one study 1 or 2 tbsps (15 or 30 milliliters) in apple cider vinegar every day for 3 months helped overweight adults shed around 2.6 and

3.7 additional pounds (1.2 and 1.7 kg) specifically.

2 tablespoons of apple cider vinegar daily are also proven to help dieters shed almost twice as much weight in three months as compared to people who didn't take in apple cider vinegar.

It is possible to mix it in a glass of water and then drink it before eating or mix it in with oil to create a salad dress.

In conjunction with other diet plans and also lifestyle adjustments, Apple cider vinegar is particularly effective in aiding weight loss.

Consuming 1 2 tablespoons (1530-ml) from apple cider vinegar daily for a few months can help improve weight control in people who are overweight.

The apple cider vinegar has become a well-known ingredient in diet plans around the world due to its fat-burning commercial or residential properties, as in addition to the health benefits. It is made up of fermented apple juice that is commonly used in dressings for salads and as food additives to boost the level of satisfaction as well as help to consume less calories. According to research, the vinegar made from apple cider is an excellent beverage to aid in weight loss, but can it be effective?

Most of the products that claim to help speed up fat-burning, such as "slim teas" as well as supplements don't work or be unsafe for commercial or residential properties that could harm your health and wellbeing.

Many slimmers claim that they have found the "wonder" device for weight loss that can help you lose weight faster.

All over the world, both genders are buying the apple cider vinegar bottle to help reduce and shed the weight.

It has been used for many years, and it has been proven to aid in the killing of bacteria and viruses and was also employed for cleaning and sanitizing, treating lice, nail fungi, the growth of ear infections and so on So is it a product that you ought to be taking?

It's been proven that taking two tablespoons each throughout the day with apple cider vinegar could create a feeling of weight and reduce the amount of food consumed during the course of the day.

In a study conducted by PubMed.gov It was discovered that drinking a few 2 tablespoons (15 or 30 milliliters) in apple cider vinegar each day for three months helped obese adults shed about 2.6 (1.2 kilograms) as well as 3.7 additional pounds (1.7 kg).

Expert in weight loss as well as the owner of the fitness blog, Carla George stated: "Two tablespoons of food a day can help people lose twice as much weight in three months as compared with those who really did not consume it at any way."

It is actually suggested that the most effective method to drink an alcohol vinegar apple cider is by mixing a few teaspoons in an ice-cold glass of water and consume it prior to eating or mix it with oil for an outfit for salads.

Weight loss of significant magnitude will be experienced when you pair apple cider vinegar with other diet plans and lifestyle changes.

Factors Apple Cider Vinegar Weight Loss Works

This isn't like the advert in the back of a book that the claim that it is not able to last. Studies have shown the fact that vinegar made from apple could provide amazing health benefits that could help you lose weight. Here's the way to do it.

Apple cider vinegar can help regulate blood sugar levels

Apple cider vinegar to lose weight could be a good option to try. The apple cider vinegar weight loss plan can affect the way blood sugar levels are controlled as per a study conducted by Carol Johnston, PhD, at Arizona State University. Explore even more remarkable health benefits and health benefits of drinking apples cider vinegar.

ACV affects exactly how food is taken up

Researchers believe that the apple cider vinegar used to lose weight can help achieve the blood sugar law by a variety of ways. "Dr. Johnston thinks the acetic acid present in the vinegar blocks disaccharidases, enzymes that break down starches to aid digestion of food and are able to be absorbed directly into bloodstream," Zuckerbrot states.

Vinegar may help individuals lose weight by increasing the sensation of volume , and also reducing the amount of food consumed during the day.

In one research study just a few tbsps (15 or 30 milliliters) in apple cider vinegar per day for 3 months helped overweight adults shed around 2.6 and 3.7 additional pounds (1.2 and 1.7 kg) specifically.

2 tablespoons of apple cider vinegar daily has also been found to assist dieters shed nearly twice the weight in three months as compared to those who didn't take the apple cider vinegar

It is possible to mix it in a glass of water and then drink it before eating or mix the oil with it to create the perfect salad dress.

In conjunction with other eating plans and ways of living changes, Apple cider vinegar is extremely effective in aiding lose weight.

Consuming 1- 2 tablespoons (1530-ml) in apple cider vinegar each day for a number of months could improve the weight loss of those who are overweight.

Apple cider vinegar can be a well-known product in the world of weight loss because of its popular weight loss building as well as benefits for health and wellbeing. The vinegar is created from fermented apple juice that is typically used in clothing for salads as well as food additives to improve satiation and also as help you consume less calories. There is evidence that Apple cider vinegar can be a great beverage to aid in weight loss, but is it really effective?

The majority of products which claim to in weight loss, such as "slim teas" and supplements do not work or could have potentially harmful components that could harm your health and well-being.

Many slimmers claim that they have found the "wonder" weight loss device that helps you shed excess weight much faster.

Everywhere in the world, males and females alike are reaching for the apple cider vinegar bottle in search of trimming and shed the stubborn weight.

The apple cider vinegar is in use for many years as well as has been proven to assist in killing viruses composed of bacteria and was commonly used to cleanse and sanitizing, treating lice, nail fungi verrucas and also ear infections. So is it a product you ought to be taking in?

It's been observed that taking 2 tablespoons each day in apple cider vinegar may increase the sensation of bulk and reduce the amount of food consumed during the day.

In a study carried out by PubMed.gov it was found that drinking 1 or 2 tablespoons (15 or 30 milliliters) in apple cider vinegar each day for three months helped overweight adults shed around 2.6 (1.2 kilograms) as well as 3.7 additional pounds (1.7 kg).

Weight loss expert and the health and fitness blog's administrator, Carla George stated: "Two daily tbsps of food can help dieters shed nearly two times the weight in three months compared with those who really didn't consume it at all."

It is actually suggested that the best way to drink an alcohol vinegar apple cider is mixing it with a few tablespoons into the water in a glass and drink it before eating dishes or mix it with oil to create an outfit for salads.

Weight loss of significant magnitude will occur when you combine apple cider vinegar along with different diet plans as well as changes to your lifestyle.

Factors Apple Cider Vinegar Weight Loss Works

This isn't like the advert in the back of a magazine that promises that it will not last. Research has proven the fact that vinegar made from apple may be a potent source of health and properties at home that could help in losing weight. Here's how.

Apple cider vinegar helps control blood sugar levels

Apple cider vinegar to lose weight could be a good option to try. A weight loss method can influence the way blood sugar is managed in accordance with a study conducted by Carol Johnston, PhD, at Arizona State University. Explore even more astonishing benefits to health and wellness using apples cider vinegar.

ACV influences the way food is consumed

Scientists believe that the use of apple cider vinegar aids in the achievement of the blood-sugar law in a number of different ways. "Dr. Johnston thinks the acid present in the vinegar hinders disaccharidases, enzymes which break down starches to aid in digestion that are taken directly into bloodstream," Zuckerbrot states.

Enhances Fullness and Lowers Calorie Intake

Apple cider vinegar could be a way to advertise the quantity, which could decrease calories consumed

In a tiny study in 11 participants, those who consumed vinegar in high-carb dishes had 55% less blood glucose reaction after one hour after eating.

They also ate 200-275 less calories throughout the day.

In addition to its effects on appetite Apple cider vinegar has also been found to decrease the rate at which food items leave your stomach.

In a different, small study that involved apple cider vinegar, eating it together with a starchy food decreased the draining of the stomach. The result was a heightened sensation of weight as well as a decrease in blood glucose levels and insulin levels

Certain people may be suffering from an issue that makes this risk unavoidable.

Gastroparesis, which is also known as postponed stomach draining, is an incredibly common issue in diabetics with type 1 problems. Because it's hard to predict how long it's going to take blood sugar levels to rise after eating, timing the intake of insulin in conjunction with food can prove to be a hassle.

Since apple cider vinegar has been found to prolong the duration of time food is still in your stomach When consumed with food, it could cause more gastroparesis.

Apple cider vinegar helps promote the volume of your body, mainly because of delayed tummy clearing. This could result in reduced calories consumed. It could result in more severe gastoparesis for certain.

It can help you lose weight and body Fat

The results of a human research study, it is clear Apple cider vinegar can have amazing effects on weight as well as body fat.

In this research study over 12 weeks in this 12-week research study, there were 144 overweight Japanese adults consumed 1 tablespoon (15 milliliters) in vinegar and 2 tablespoons (30 milliliters) of vinegar, or an alcohol-based sugar pill on a regular basis.

They were advised to reduce their consumption of alcohol however otherwise follow their normal diet plan and work throughout the study.

People who consumed 1 tablespoon (15 milliliters) of vinegar a day hadtypically benefits that correlated with:

- Weight loss: 2.6 extra pounds (1.2 kg).

A decrease in the body fat percentage: 0.7%.

A decrease in waistline: 0.5 in (1.4 centimeters).

Triglycerides - Reduce in triglycerides 26 percent.

This is the result of people who consume 2 tablespoons (30 mg) of vinegar every day:.

- Weight loss: 3.7 extra pounds (1.7 kg).

Reduced body fat percentage: 0.9%.

Reduced waistline: 0.75 in (1.9 centimeters).

Triglycerides - Reduced 26 percent.

The sugar pill team actually got 0.9 grams (0.4 kgs) as well as their midsection area was slightly larger.

Based on this study according to this research, adding 1 or 2 tablespoons in apple cider vinegar into your diet plan can help in losing weight. It may also reduce your body fat content as well as help your belly slimmer and reduce blood triglycerides.

It is one of a handful of human studies that have looked into the effects of vinegar on weight loss. The study was quite extensive and, while the results are encouraging further research studies are needed.

Furthermore, a six-week study conducted on mice fed a high-fat diet high in calories found that the team with high dose vinegar received 10% lower in fat than control group in addition to 2% smaller in weight than the vinegar-low dose team. In one study, overweight participants who used 1-2 tbsp (1530 to 30 ml) in apple cider vinegar each day for 12 weeks, lost weight as well as body fat.

ACV may help control cravings.

Consuming this superfood could end your food cravings and make you feel great. "Acetic acid, which is the main component of vinegar, is touted as a natural hunger suppressant" Zuckerbrot states.

ACV affects the insulin guideline.

You should be eating bread after the completion of your meal for the exact reason that you should begin your meal by drinking apple cider vinegar to lower insulin levels. "It appears in the findings of a tiny study published within The American Diabetes Association journal, Diabetes Care, that eating vinegar alongside a carbohydrate-rich food may increase insulin sensitiveness," Palinski-Wade explains.

ACV could help in losing fat.

Does apple cider vinegar help to melt the extra weight? Zuckerbrot cites an earlier study that examined the effects of consumption of apple cider vinegar on body weight and belly fat in overweight 175 Japanese subjects.

ACV could increase metabolic rate.

Apple cider vinegar could be the trick if you wish to increase your metabolic rate. "Although this has not been proven in research on human studies, a pet study that was conducted in Japan discovered that consumption of vinegar may increase the production of an enzyme that is responsible of fat loss" Palinski-Wade says. If you drink apple cider vinegar on a regular basis try ACV and get yourself prepared for any issues that may happen for your body.

Apple cider vinegar for weight loss

Here are some benefits that apple cider vinegar has, making it ideal for weight loss:

1. A reduced calorie beverage

About 100 grams of ACV have approximately 22 calories. This means it's beverages that are low in calories that could aid in weight loss. Incorporating a tablespoon of ACV into the glass of water, and drinking alcohol at the beginning of the morning can help to melt off belly fat.

2. Helps to reduce the accumulation of fat

In the study published by the journal Bioscience, Biotechnology and also Biochemistry, acetic acid which is the principal component of vinegar, was discovered to lower the amount of fat in studies on pets. The scientists' group also studied the results of overweight Japanese in a double-blind study. Additionally, daily drinking apple cider vinegar can aid in the prevention of metabolic disorders by reducing excess weight.

3. It helps you stay fuller for a longer period of time.

A study published by The Journal of Clinical Nutrition discovered the acetic acid present in ACV can make you feel fuller for a longer period of time, thus keeping you from eating too much or having cravings. This can help in consuming less calories and will result in actual weight loss on the range.

4. Handles blood glucose degrees

Research studies suggest apple cider vinegar helps to maintain blood sugar levels especially after eating an item that is high in carbs. A stable blood glucose level is crucial to ensure a healthy and and balanced fat burning.

How can you make the most from apple cider vinegar to aid in weight loss?

Do not consume apple cider vinegar just as it is. Instead reduce the strength of the remedy with water to ensure that you are not consuming a large amount of acid.

It is possible to use it to dress up your salad made of olive oil for the long-term reduction in weight.

It is recommended to distribute the use by taking 2 to 3 doses throughout the day. Additionally, it is advised to drink ACV alcohol prior to eating meals.

Although a few times a week in the form of vinegar made from apple could be safe, frequent usage could alter the excellent results because ACV is extremely acidic. If you consume it frequently or in large quantities it could cause irritation to your throat.

In the final hours of the day, drinking an apple cider vinegar can be found to help reduce weight as well as provide a number of other health benefits.

Different varieties of vinegar could provide similar benefits, but those with less acetic acid content might have less powerful impact.

Chapter 12: Improved Digestion

A lot of people drink apple cider vinegar prior to protein-rich meals to improve digestion.

The theory is the apple cider vinegar raises the acidity level in your stomach, which helps your body to develop more pepsin, an enzyme which breaks down healthy proteins.

While there's no research to support the use of vinegar in digestion of food, other acidic supplements, like betaine HCL can significantly increase the acidity in the stomach.

Acidic foods such as apple cider vinegar could yield similar results, but there is a lot of research is needed.

The people who use apple cider vinegar to aid in digestion of food usually consume 1 two tablespoons (15to 30 milliliters) along with an instant glass of water before meals, however there's no evidence that supports the dosage.

There are insurance policies that claim that alcohol consumption of 1 to 2 tablespoons (1530-ml) from apple cider vinegar prior to eating helps digestion. There is currently no research to support this practice.

No matter how it's advertised regardless of how it's advertised, apple cider vinegar isn't an all-purpose remedy, but it contains elements that could be beneficial for digestion of food. Ask your physician about the advantages and disadvantages of adding apple cider vinegar in your diet.

The Prebiotic

Apple cider vinegar is thought of to be a prebiotic, do not be misled by probiotics, like yogurt. Yogurt is one of the a source of these pleasant bacteria. Prebiotics provide food to beneficial germs, and help to preserve the number of bacteria in your intestine while as well as keeping your gastrointestinal system healthy and well-balanced. Prebiotics such as apple cider vinegar may also assist in boosting calcium absorption.

Easy-to-Digest Carb

Apples are thought of as to be a food with high levels of FODMAP. A cider of apples is considered to be a food with low levels of FODMAPs.

Tooth Erosion

A 2012 study of situation research document published within The Dutch Magazine for Dentistry kept in mind that the consumption of apple cider vinegar could cause destruction in tooth enamel. Consuming American Dental Association-approved sugar-free periodontal after you drink or consume drinks that have vinegar from apple cider can help shield your teeth from harm caused due to an acidic flavor.

Include ACV in a balanced and balanced diet plan

There are many ways to incorporate ACV in a healthy and balanced diet. Certain people drink ACV containing alcohol straight, however some prefer to mix the drink with water, or other fluids.

To benefit from the many benefits of ACV Consider drinking around 1 tbsp or two times per day.

When purchasing ACV make sure you purchase an ACV brand name that contains "the mother." It is an enveloping layer that is made by yeast, and bacteria that produce acetic acids. It grows normally during the fermentation process.

The layer is removed from the typical vinegars, however it's also an antbiotic (advertising the growth of balanced and healthy microorganisms that live in your digestive tract) and is also an array of beneficial microorganisms.

Prior to drinking alcohol raw vinegar that has not been filtered, shake it vigorously to distribute the mother. Add 1 to 2 tablespoons in 1 mug of water.

Here are some other ways to incorporate ACV into your daily routine:

Create ACV tea. Add 1 tbsp ACV to 1 cup of boiling water.

Incorporate ACV into a smoothie mix. It is possible to disguise the bitter taste of ACV by adding it in a healthy fruit smoothie. To maintain a balanced and healthy digestion, place 1 tablespoon of ACV, 1/2 cup of raspberries and 1/3 cup of apple pieces as well as half of a banana in a food processor or blender with an ice cube.

ACV creates a delicious salad-inspired clothing. For an easy and fast outfit mix 1 tablespoon of ACV with 1 tablespoon of olive oil.

Apple CIDER VINEGAR Need help with BLOATING?

The apple cider vinegar advocates offer a variety of claims regarding its health and wellness benefits. One such claim is that drinking one tablespoon of apple cider vinegar mixed with a glass of warm water could help with the bloating issue and many other digestive problems.

Natural home remedies made with the use Apple cider vinegar (ACV) to address intestinal tract issues has become popular in the present time. Although there is no evidence which proves ACV can treat the bloating issue, but there are some unscientific statements that claim it's valid. Studies have also shown that ACV offers a variety of other benefits due to its natural properties.

Keep reading to learn additional information about the benefits and dangers of ACV for the bloating and other therapies that could help in reducing the symptoms.

What causes the cause of bloating?

Bloating is the accumulation of gas in the stomach or the intestinal tracts. Gas production is a common component of both eating as well as food digestion, but it can trigger discomfort in certain circumstances that include:

The body has excess fat the body.

There is plenty of it

It occurs within the upper of the intestinal tract in contrast to the colon

If they've got a full with balloons of air in their stomach or have tension in their intestinal tracts, and also a decrease in abdominal regions, a person could feel.

The reason for this could be due to:

Consuming far too much

Consuming as fast as you can

Consuming food that are difficult for the body to absorb. taking in

germs that move to the small intestine, for example in the small intestinal tract, microbes that are growth (SIBO).

Sometimes, gas might signify various other problems, such as irregular bowel movements or a persistent problem, such as cranky digestive tract disorder (IBS).

When germs ferment carbohydrates in food, the body creates 2 primary gases. These gases are methane as well as hydrogen. Study has actually connected greater quantities of methane gas with a number of digestion problems, consisting of irregularity, IBS, and also excessive weight.

There is no straight treatment for bloating. Rather, the body has a tendency to pass the gas with time, which lowers the pain.

Some therapies might assist manage the signs or aid the gas pass quicker, yet bloating might return if individuals do not deal with the underlying reason.

Does ACV aid with bloating?

Apple cider vinegar has actually come to be a prominent natural remedy for digestion concerns generally. One idea is that ACV is a reliable as well as fast treatment for bloating. There is extremely little straight proof to back this certain case.

ACV might assist in particular circumstances. ACV is normally acidic, therefore for individuals with reduced belly level of acidity, utilizing ACV might assist increase tummy acid degrees to help food digestion. Theoretically, this might avoid gas as well as bloating, which a sluggish food digestion can create.

ACV is additionally an antimicrobial material, suggesting it might aid eliminate microorganisms in the belly or intestinal tracts. Excess germs or germs in the top intestinal tracts launch gases that might cause bloating, so ACV might aid with signs and symptoms.

Just how to utilize ACV for bloating.

There is restricted clinical proof that ACV aids with bloating, individuals might desire to attempt it to see if it relieves their signs and symptoms.

Making use of ACV for bloating is easy. Including a tbsp of ACV to a tiny glass of cozy water and afterwards consuming it prior to or after a dish or when an individual really feels puffed up is all they require to do.

A variety of beverages, salad dressings, and also various other foods additionally consist of ACV that might assist to ease signs of bloating.

Some individuals that do not take pleasure in the preference might select to take ACV pills. It is essential to consume alcohol a big glass of water with these pills to ensure they get to the belly.

It is best to utilize raw, unfiltered, natural ACV. This all-natural kind of ACV includes hairs of yeast and also germs that provide the vinegar a somewhat over cast appearance. Unfiltered ACV might additionally have trace element, healthy proteins, as well as enzymes that are missing in filteringed system ACV.

Shake up the vinegar prior to gauging it to catch these yeasts as well as germs. Filteringed system ACV will certainly look practically clear in contrast, also after drinking.

APPLE CIDER VINEGAR FOR HAIR

Apple cider vinegar (ACV) is a popular health food and condiment. It is made from apples using a method of fermentation which enriches it with live cultures, minerals, and acids.

As a home remedy, ACV has many uses. One of these is to improve scalp quality as a hair wash, reinforce hair, and increase visibility.

While being praised as a home "panacea" and "cure-all" for health problems despite being under-researched, the benefits and evidence behind ACV have when it comes to hair care.

Apple cider vinegar can be an excellent natural treatment for those struggling with hair issues such as itchy scalp and hair breakage.

Why use ACV to take care of the hair?

For why this popular beauty condiment is right for your body, there are many reasons.

Acidity and pH

In addition to having some well-researched medical effects, apple cider vinegar is an acidic product for one. This contains the right acetic acid concentrations.

Hair that appears weak, dry, and frizzy on the pH scale seems to be more alkaline and lower. The theory is that an acid material, such as ACV, helps lower pH and returns to improve hair quality.

Antimicrobial

Also, a standard home disinfectant is antimicrobial ACV. It can help control the bacteria and fungus that can cause problems with scalp and hair, such as mild infections and itchiness.

Other claims

Many reasons Apple cider vinegar, including vitamin C and B, is lauded for being high in hair-friendly vitamins and minerals. Some also argue that it contains alpha-hydroxy acid that helps exfoliate the skin of the scalp and that it is anti-inflammatory that can help with dandruff.

How do I use hair care for ACV?

It can be done quickly to clean an ACV.

Mix with just a few teaspoons of apple cider vinegar.

Give the mixture evenly over your hair between shampooing and washing, operating in your scalp.

Let it rest for a few minutes.

Rinse clean.

Coconuts and Kettlebells consider adding in the solution a few drops of essential oil if the acid taste is too intense for you. Upon rinsing, also, the smell should go away quickly.

Try to incorporate the wash a few days a week into your hair care routine. You can also increase the amount of ACV you use when cleaning or rinsing. It is generally recommended to carry it about five teaspoons or less.

Eight Ways Apple Cider Vinegar Can Benefit Your Hair

It could potentially help ward off dandruff

"Apple cider vinegar has antibacterial and antifungal effects," said board-certified dermatologist Dr. Debra Jaliman. "Fungus is what induces dandruff.[ACV] contains malic acid that helps to keep the pH level of the scalp stable. Dandruff is an accumulation on the scalp, which happens when too much yeast is present in oily areas of the skin. Using a solution of ACV can help prevent this build-up on the scalp called dandruff." "It is helpful in the treatment of dandruff because it allows lower levels of skin yeast.

These same properties can help with product build-up

Although they may seem the same thing, dandruff is different from soap build-up, which can occur when we less often wash our hair and rely on items such as dry shampoo to last longer between washes.

Styling products that leave stains in the hair, but as Dr. Jaliman says, apple cider vinegar is "an alpha hydroxy acid that helps exfoliate the body. It also has a skin-like pH, which helps maintain a healthy pH equilibrium between the skin and scalp," potentially helping to clear the locks after days of gels, mousses, and sprays.

"ACV is somewhat acidic," said the board-certified dermatologist Erum Ilyas, MD, MBE, FAAD, based in Pennsylvania. "Our skin is also naturally acidic from the oils and sebum from our scalp. Hair products also interact with the pH balance in our cosmetics. If our hair becomes healthy or mildly acidic, the cuticle becomes smooth. Once we apply hair products, many of them bind to our hair by expanding the skin slightly and making the hair more alkaline.

Try apple cider vinegar to ease scalp itchiness

There are several explanations why you may feel scalp scratching, ranging from dandruff to medical conditions such as atopic dermatitis and psoriasis, and others. While you should certainly check in with the doctor and dermatologist for any excessive scratching, Dr. Jaliman said that ACV could help alleviate some of the itchiness, explaining that "Apple cider vinegar helps rebalance the pH of your skin. Balancing your scalp's pH can help reduce itchiness."

ACV might help prevent hair loss and stimulate new hair growth

Adding apple cider vinegar to your hair care regimen "will help keep your skin clean by avoiding infection and maintaining a stable pH rate," Dr. Jaliman said, adding that "this will encourage hair growth. ACV softly exfoliates the scalp, which in effect will facilitate hair growth and cleaner hair."

ACV might help prevent hair loss and stimulate new hair growth

Adding apple cider vinegar to your hair care regimen "can help keep your scalp clean by avoiding infection and keeping a stable pH rate," Dr. Jaliman said, adding that "this will encourage hair growth. ACV gently exfoliates the scalp and, in effect, can facilitate hair growth and healthier skin."

It can help make the hair feel sleek, gentle and light

 because we know the toiletries and ingredients, as well as exposure to the elements, tends to roughen the cuticula of our hair, we are often left with strings that look dull and twisted.

"Apple cider vinegar can help close the cuticle of the skin," Dr. Jaliman said. "The hair will turn out to be more stable and much healthier. ACV helps remove hair buildup," which will also improve visibility.

These benefits can help prevent split ends and breakage

Just as ACV tends to close the cuticula of the scalp, it works to keep the hair healthy overall, which can assist with damage and split ends, Dr. Ilyas said, although this is not a miracle cure.

"Occasionally, using ACV can add acidity to the hair follicle, smoothing the cuticula and making it less stiff. By doing so in practice, you may be able to prevent split ends and breakage."

ACV might help restore hair's natural texture

While it's not a cure-all for all of your hair woes, adding apple cider vinegar to your hair care routine can help restore the natural texture of your hair after harm from equipment, products, and environmental stressors, said Kathleen Cook Suozzi, MD, assistant professor at Yale School of Medicine's Department of Dermatology. She told INSIDER that "ACV can help smooth hair strands through the alpha hydroxy acids it provides. By removing dead skin cells and dirt, AHAs exfoliate the skin." "Likewise, it can help exfoliate and smooth hair strands.

It might help ward off certain scalp infections

You must check-in with the physician, as with any medical concern, but our experts say apple cider vinegar may be helpful for certain diseases of the scalp.

"ACV has antimicrobial properties completely, so it can be an active method of preventing some scalp infections," Dr. Ilyas said. "Medical studies have been told to try to support the widespread use of ACV. At maximum doses, ACV is topically active against bacteria, yeast, and fungus. Moreover, if concentrated, it tends to retain its potency against bacteria at a concentration of 25%, but it lacks effectiveness against yeast and fungi." "And, depending on the source of the scalp disease, it may fire.

Things to watch out for

It's all about bringing hair back into balance using apple cider vinegar. It may be overdone if you're not patient. Instead, if your hair or scalp problems get worse, stop using ACV. Or, try to lower your rinse amount or the frequency you use it.

Apple cider vinegar contains recognized caustic acetic acids. It ensures that the skin can be scratched and burnt.

When adding ACV directly to the body, it is often diluted with water. If your rinses are too substantial, try to dilute it more — but it almost always clears up within a few days when discomfort occurs.

Even avoid eye contact. If touch happens, flush off easily with air.

Pursue the above instructions, and it may be considered entirely safe to use apple cider vinegar.

Apple Cider Vinegar Hair Rinse

When there seems to be a lot out there, the thought of using an apple cider vinegar hair rinse— you're not alone.

I was a little doubtful, to say the least when I applied an apple cider vinegar hair wash to my routine (using that pure apple cider vinegar). The last thing I wanted to do was wander around with a sour vinegar head with apple cider.

Yet I first ditched my traditional toner for a DIY apple cider vinegar facial toner after doing a lot of research on the effects of apple cider vinegar for hair and skin and was blown away with the results. Moving into a more natural skincare routine changed my skin's appearance completely, and since I made the switch, my face has been free of any significant pimples, blemishes, and acne.

One of the many things people tend to ignore is their pH levels of hair and sebum. Sebum is the natural oil that your scalp produces.

The potential for hydrogen, also known as pH, must range from 4.5 to 5.5. If your pH is not within that range, it can cause your hair to fall off, get dry, and encourage your scalp to expand with fungi and bacteria.

You can control the pH levels in your skin by using many of the items and shops available, and even some of the DIY tools you may use.

I decided to experiment with an apple cider vinegar skin wash soon afterward. Apple cider vinegar is now one of my favorite ways to keep up with my skin and hair. And while apple cider vinegar has many advantages—both externally and topically, this apple cider vinegar hair rinse is one of my favorite applications.

Why does a hair wash with Apple Cider Vinegar?

To give you enough faith to pour on your head this apple cider vinegar hair wash, it is vital that you know the fundamentals about how the hairs on your head come into being.

What we usually see as "hair" is a two-part structure composed of a follicle, a tunnel-like section in the body, and a shaft, the recognizable component which rises above the surface.

There are sebaceous glands just below the skin surface that secrete sebum through the hair follicle. This oil lubricates hair and skin and is part of the acid mantle, a fragile, slightly acidic product that preserves and prevents hair and skin's overall health. The acid mantle is also essential to the quality of our body, which is crucial to most of us. The shaft's outer layer is compromised by tightly packed overlapping scales, commonly known as the cuticle. The acid mantle is influential in the flatness of cuticular scales, which gives skin a bright, smooth look and protects against lack of moisture.

Unfortunately, it is easy to disrupt this system, which is the leading cause of the ever-popular bad hair day. Usually, the acid mantle has a pH of about 5, indicating it is slightly acidic. Many hair care products, treatments, and shampoos are more alkaline (have a pH above 7), which can contaminate the acid mantle or remove it.

When the mantle with acid is alkaline, the skin swells, and the scales open on the cuticle, leaving it vulnerable to crack. It also results in frizzy, brittle hair with a "dull" appearance because instead of reflecting it, the hair absorbs light. (Perfect for photo day!) Other causes, including stress, diet, and sweat, may also interrupt the acid mantle. Therefore, it is essential for stable, healthy hair to proactively return our hair to its normal pH and preserve the acid mantle.

Why the raw of Apple Cider Vinegar?

Apple cider vinegar raw (or unfiltered) is simply the by-product of apple fermentation. Apples are loaded with potassium, pectin, malic acid, and calcium, and bubbling with even more beneficial acids and enzymes fortify the end product. Fresh apple cider vinegar preserves all the nutrients in the liquid, which is why it is compared over pasteurized vinegar apple cider.

Since apple cider vinegar has a pH of about 3 (meaning it is acidic), it helps balance the pH of the skin when correctly mixed with steam, resulting in many good hair days.

Apple Cider Vinegar Hair Rinse Benefits

Although there is no formal research exploring the benefits of a hair rinse of apple cider vinegar, Based on the characteristics of apple cider vinegar, there are many positive side effects you can encounter. Apple cider vinegar provides nutrients that produce luscious locks, including vitamins B, vitamin C, and potassium.

Because it is very acidic, it also tends to maintain the acid mantle's normal pH. Exposure to this acidity strengthens the outer layer of the skin and flattens the cuticle, resulting in comfortably smooth hair, "slides," and less susceptible to tangling and snagging.

Apple cider vinegar also includes organic alpha-hydroxy acid, which softly exfoliates the scalp and body, allowing the elimination and build-up of dead skin cells from sweat or traditional hair products. It improves the hair's look, eliminates itchiness, and enables enhanced styling.

Apple cider vinegar can provide relief for those suffering scalp-related conditions such as dandruff due to it's anti-viral, anti-fungal, and anti-bacterial properties. Apple cider vinegar is also anti-inflammatory in addition to being antimicrobial, which can prevent the usual skin irritation with dandruff and a sore, flaky scalp.

Another common problem with which an apple cider vinegar rinse can help is to build up the product. Many shampoos cannot clean and clarify to remove all products from your hair thoroughly.

With time, it causes it to build up, making the hair feel filthy. It doesn't just feel gross, but it can hinder your hair growth. Products start clogging the pores on your scalp over time, stopping hair from emerging out of them.

While it prevents oil build-up, dandruff will also be eliminated by the wash, and an itchy scalp will be relieved. Apple cider vinegar rinses also contain the potent antibacterial and antifungal agents that stop dandruff and hair loss.

Use apple cider vinegar in your shampoo, and adding it to a soothing hair mask can minimize friction and decrease the porosity of your skin, making it feel smoother and allowing more structure for curly hair. If you're afraid that washing your hair with vinegar apple cider shampoo would make it taste like vinegar, you can add a little drop of essential oil to the formula, but generally, the scent will disappear once it's dry.

If you decide to go for apple cider vinegar, you can either go with a well-known brand like Bragg's or choose another one. It is essential to ensure that the vinegar is not pure, as this ensures that most of its properties, such as antibacterial enzymes, have been filtered. Alternatively, consider one in white, raw, or unfiltered, sunny.

It is quick to use a wash with apple cider vinegar as a hair treatment. Rinse it with 1⁄4 apple cider vinegar and 3⁄4 water after washing your hair.

Let it flow from your scalp to the ends of your hair and rub it in your scalp. Then wash the vinegar with water and leave a bit of the rinse in your hair to make it easier to remove. You will almost immediately begin to see the effects.

And the best part of that? All these benefits come at a very affordable price.

Apple Cider Vinegar Hair Rinse

Ingredients

• 2-4 tbsp raw apple cider vinegar

• 16 oz cool water

• 1-2 drops lavender oil (optional)

Directions

Blend apple cider vinegar, steam, and essential oil (optional) in a plastic bottle after shampooing and rinsing the hair. Pour the rinse over your whole scalp, tipping your head back, allowing the paste to flow through your body. Be careful to avoid eye contact. Let the mixture settle for 1-2 minutes on your skin. Then, thoroughly rinse.

Tips and tricks

1.   Depending on your individual needs, the specific amount of apple cider vinegar you need will vary. If you don't see success with the lower ratio, I recommend starting with 2 tbsp and working your way up to 4 tbsp.

2.   Usually, dry hair will do better with less apple cider vinegar as a general rule of thumb, while those with wet hair and scalp issues like dandruff will do better with more apple cider vinegar.

3.   It will depend on your current hair and scalp situation to determine how often to apply this rinse. I consider once a week adding this wash. If you have dry or weak skin, only 1-2 days a month may be best for you to rinse your hair. Experiment to see for yourself what works best. A good starting point is once a week.

4.   The best way to consistently incorporate this apple cider vinegar skin wash is to blend it in a plastic squeeze bottle right before you get into the shower. Then take the bottle in the tub with you and wash your hair after shampooing.

5.   It won't smell like apple cider vinegar anymore after you rinse the apple cider vinegar and your hair dries.

6.   You may reduce your overall rinse by half if your hair is shoulder length or shorter. You are using 1 cup of cold water and 1-2 tbsp of vinegar for apple cider.

7.   You don't have to use a traditional conditioner after the apple cider vinegar skin wash, as the vinegar solution will automatically condition the body. When you find that the absence of conditioner seems to affect the look of your hair after some experiments, I recommend applying conditioner to the ends of your hair after the wash.

Chapter 13: Apple Cider Vinegar For Skin

Perhaps the secret to good complexion is sitting in your cupboard! Use skin apple cider vinegar that will make you look younger years.

Apple cider vinegar is an excellent treatment for the symptoms with warts, pimples, acne, and other hair. Furthermore, preserving and enhancing your skin's overall health is a great everyday product: it can make your skin look younger and feel cleaner.

Apple cider vinegar, or ACV, is a natural remedy that contains no harsh chemical substances. It is a skin care method that is tried and preferred over many centuries.

Apple cider vinegar's versatile wonders have been making the mainstream rounds in recent years. In addition to its varied and delicious uses in the kitchen, many people drink apple cider vinegar alone or diluted with water to help digestive health (thanks to good bacteria that your gut loves) and even regulate blood sugar (studies have found improving insulin function).

But the benefits of apple cider vinegar inside the body are just the beginning; for a wide range of skin, scalp, and hair benefits, it is also used topically. Seriously, with this stuff, people swear to improve all kinds of skin issues, from skin dullness to acne scars and age spots. And it's not just another new skincare fad: "Apple cider vinegar (ACV) has been used for thousands of years as a natural remedy," says Rachele Cochran Gathers, MD, a dermatologist certified board member.

Apple cider vinegar is an ingredient that has many benefits for both the health and the skin. Rich in acetic, citric, malic, and amino acid, it also contains vitamins, enzymes, and mineral salts that are beneficial to your skin.

This comes with numerous skin-related issues when summer begins. As sun heat on our skin becomes very harsh and results in many skin-related problems such as sunburn, suntan, acne, pimples, spots, and other skin infections. Protecting our bodies from these things becomes very complicated for us. So here we are with an ingredient you can easily find in your kitchens that can do amazing things for your body. Apple cider vinegar is an ingredient that has many uses for both the body and the skin. High in acetic, citric, malic, and amino acid, it also includes vitamins, enzymes, and mineral salts that are helpful to your body.

Apple cider vinegar (ACV) is essentially a magic elixir— from improving weight loss to diabetes treatment, it feels like there's nothing ACV can't do.

It can also do good for your body if used correctly.

Apple cider vinegar can have antibacterial, anti-fungal, and antiviral effects in general. However, the use of ACV on the skin must be careful, as it can cause significant irritation when applied topically without dilution, leading to burns or blisters. It's an acid, after all. And while it is widely available, most concentrations may be too powerful to apply without diluting it to your skin. So you shouldn't just slather it from the bottle straight.

But first, why should we be worried about our skin's health? For one, it performs several vital functions, including:

•   Body temperature control.

•   They are protecting us from adverse environmental factors.

•   You are receiving and transmitting external stimulation information.

The protection of the body should, therefore, be part of any effort to maintain a healthy lifestyle. Read on to discover how apple cider vinegar will help if you want to improve your skin's health.

Common Uses of Apple Cider Vinegar for Skin

"Many claim that ACV can help[alleviate] eczema and acne, fade fine lines, and make skin look brighter and more youthful," says Gathers. "People use it as a skin toner and to help treat acne-prone areas." However, Dr. Gathers warns that these statements are purely anecdotal, despite the number of people who have fallen in love with it. "There is no good scientific study to prove ACV's claims for skin healing," she says. "I would advise that your dermatologist test you first before switching to ACV."

Why exactly does Apple Cider Vinegar Help Skin?

Its composition can be beneficial to skin in many ways. ACV has antibacterial and antimicrobial properties and can help kill skin bacteria and yeast associated with conditions such as acne, eczema, and dandruff. The high acidity level of ACV may also improve many skin conditions (but note well: its high acidity makes water dilution necessary). "Healthy skin lies on the acid end of the pH spectrum to get a little technical. Individuals with eczema, though, may have an elevated skin pH that can weaken the skin barrier and make it more susceptible to infection. Because ACV is acidic, it can help restore some of the normal ph. of the body. ACV is also desired for more specific beauty qualities in addition to treating more problematic skin conditions. This includes citric acid, an alpha hydroxyl acid (or AHA) used to exfoliate, brighten, and smooth[your teint], as well as polyphenolic antioxidants, which may further improve the appearance of the body.

How to Learn If it's healthy to use on your body

Before jumping right into your skin or applying an apple cider vinegar toner and soaking to your skincare regimen, learn this: ACV isn't a cure-all and may not be for everyone. "While it may be beneficial to the skin issues of some people, it is important to know that there have been no clear studies to support people's claims about using ACV as a skin treatment," Gathers says. Consult with your dermatologist at all times first. ACV is acidic, and cases of people with extreme skin irritation have been documented and even burns on the skin using it.

Check it first Always do a spot check on a separate region (think: under your jawline) before swiping it all over your face.

9 Ways Apple Cider Vinegar Can Give You Happy, Healthy Skin

Apple cider vinegar has become one of the natural skin care's darlings. Can you blame anyone for risking looking like a salad dressing if it means better skin and supposed benefits such as a cleaner, clearer skin? In the pursuit of fashion, they have done weirder stuff. The skincare experts agree that you can do great things for your body with this fermented water.

- Great spot treatment

- Helps your routine masking work better

- Helps balance your skin

- Great for hyperpigmentation

- Helps stimulate circulation

- Great DIY mask

- Improves your skin's pH

- Great for hyperpigmentation

- Great for dandruff removal

How To Make Apple Cider Vinegar Toner For Glowing Skin

Raw Organic Apple Cider Vinegar (ACV) is of great benefit to our health and body. Beneficial ingredients in fresh apple cider vinegar allow it to feel better, look better, and feel energized. It's good for skin that's susceptible to acne. I'll share the benefits and my Homemade apple cider vinegar toner experience.

It is made from healthy, organically grown apples and preserves some beneficial components as it does not pasteurize raw apple cider vinegar. ACV undergoes two processes of fermentation in which it produces enzymes and gives life to nutrients that make apple cider vinegar the powerhouse it is. Next, we will learn about apple cider vinegar's skin effects.

Apple cider vinegar toner skin benefits

•   Apple has potassium, which is one of the reasons that many people are suffering from dry skin due to potassium deficiency. Potassium keeps the skin internally moisturized and hydrated.

•   Apple pectin helps to counter age-related changes in the skin system.

•   Apple malic acid acts as an exfoliant to help remove dead skin cells, dark spots, bruises, and acne from the body.

•   Apple's skin advantages include cell regeneration, lipid barrier function, and DNA antioxidant defense.

•   Apple cider vinegar contains lactic acid, and another study has been conducted to demonstrate that lactic acid treats and prevents acne.

• Apple ash normalizes the pH of the skin.

• Apple acetic acid helps to exfoliate and moisturize the skin.

homemade apple cider vinegar toner

I've been using a combination of apple cider vinegar and water as a toner for the past three months, every night, and every evening after I wash my face. In just a few months, I saw a drastic change and improvement in my hair.

I noticed my skin tone was softer, and I had fewer dry and itchy red patches, plus less oiliness in my troubled area. On my cheeks and nose, I can see increasingly noticeable tiny pores that always seemed to be there. I have witnessed fewer frequent breakouts daily. I found that many of my past breakouts seemed to have been triggered by clogged pores and no matter how much I cleaned my head, I would still have the question, this toner was the solution I was looking for.

Substitute Water With Other Ingredients In Apple Cider Vinegar Toner

Substitute water for red wine as it gives the skin a soothing glow while eliminating tannins and blemishes. A wine's anti-aging qualities make it even more desirable. With the addition of witch hazel, green tea, essential oils such as tea tree oil or lavender, you can also customize your toner.

Also, you can replace water with cucumber juice as it will give the skin a cooling effect. For added benefits, you can also infuse the water with some fresh herbs such as basil leaves, mint leaves, oregano, neem leaves, etc. Chop some fresh herbs, bring them to a boil with water and cook for 20 minutes over low heat. Strain the mixture and allow the liquid to cool before applying it to your toner mixture instead of regular water. This boiling water can be stored in the fridge for 6-7 days in an airtight container.

How to Make Apple Cider Vinegar Toner

Ingredients

• 	Apple Cider Vinegar

- Distilled water

- Sprinkle bottle directions

How to Prepare and Use

- Pour into a glass jar, tube or bowl one portion of Natural Raw Apple Cider Vinegar.

- Use two purified or filtered water elements.

- Shake the solution with the bottle.

- Use a cotton ball or pad to add the toner to your newly cleansed body, avoiding the eye area.

- Once the apple cider vinegar toner has dried, add the usual daily moisturizer.

- Play with the ACV-to-water proportions and see what the skin likes and is most sensitive to. Once you spot it, you'll know.

Notes

- Be sure to use a pure, unfiltered apple cider vinegar with the' mom' ideally.

- Apple cider vinegar tastes like feet a bit. Once the toner dries on your face, I think the smell dissipates almost completely. Instead of letting the mixture dry on your face and staying there, try allowing it dry a bit, rinse your face quickly with a splash or two of water before applying your moisturizer if the smell does bother you too much.

• Any open pores, scratches, pimples will be stung. It's normal to break out of the apple cider vinegar. It removes evil seeds. It seems to work by purging the contaminants of your body before it begins to recover. Purging, in the case of acne, may occur.

• ACV is very acidic or 3.0 pH. Using this more than twice a day can be too much for certain types of skin, particularly if the skin has issues already.

• This functions for many, but it can be a challenge for others. And check the skin carefully to see the effects.

• New photos have been changed, but it's the same formula.

Cleanse Pores

Apple cider vinegar is particularly useful as it is an astringent component in toners as it helps control oil and decrease pores' appearance.

This deep pore cleansing clay mask flavored with vinegar from apple cider may be the solution to your acne woes. One of my favorite acne-busting, mega pore drying go-to masks is bentonite and apple cider vinegar cream.

I finally found a drug that worked after years of persistent acne, multiple medications, and many skincare options available.

Pores are tiny skin holes, each holding a follicle of hair. Genetics or oily skin condition usually causes large pores. The presence of large open pores is troubling as this means that the surface of the skin is even more vulnerable to bacteria and other pollutants. It also makes the coverage of the makeup appear sloppy and may even make the skin resistant to making-up.

The only way to keep the pores in balance is to follow a strict CTM regimen and use constant pore mitigating solutions such as primers, oils, mists, etc. But yet, the truth is still not enough for most of us who suffer from large open pores. So guarantee that your skin is toned and healthy, you need to go the extra mile. Luckily for you, this skin woe has a natural product that is the ultimate fast fix.

Add apple cider vinegar to your beauty routine and enjoy the pore-shrinking properties that it has to bring along with other skin benefits.

There are many antibacterial effects of Apple cider vinegar. This unblocks pores, eliminating bacteria, wastewater, and other contaminants from them. It also regulates the skin's pH level. This natural product includes alpha-hydroxy acids that improve cell turnover, decrease wrinkles, shorten, and tighten pores.

Directions

Combine ten tablespoons of water with two teaspoons of apple cider vinegar and pass the solution into a spray bottle to enjoy the advantages. Upon washing your head, use this solution as a toner and follow up with a moisturizer. Sprinkle this mist on your face at any time of day to clean your skin and polished your pores.

What you need for Apple Cider Vinegar Mask Bentonite Clay+:

Let's get to the good stuff now! To get going, you only need two simple ingredients and a few quick things from your kitchen to find supplies.

You're going to need:

• 1 tsp Bentonite Clay

• 1 tsp Apple Cider Vinegar (with mom)

• 1 tsp of distilled water (optional)

• One ceramic, wooden or plastic cup (preferably metal)

• One plastic or wooden spoon

• One face mask comb (included in our facial clay assortment)

What is Apple Cider Vinegar "with the mother"?

Bentonite + Apple Cider Vinegar Mask Recipe 2 You can quickly tell the difference between "with the mom" and one without an apple cider vinegar. A vinegar without apple cider is transparent, and you can see through it virtually. A mother's apple cider vinegar, my preference being Bragg Apple Cider Vinegar above, is turbid, often with sand at the base.

This includes protein strings, proteins, and helpful bacteria, all of which are the vinegar's most valuable components for apple cider. So if you purchase a product without the parent, a large part of the nutrients will be stretched.

Because that protein, enzyme, and friendly bacteria strands settle down at the bottom, be sure to give the bottle a good shake before use.

I How to Mix Bentonite Clay

In a small glass mixing bowl, add 1 tsp of clay with 1 tsp of apple cider vinegar and 1 tsp of liquid with a plastic spoon or mini spatula. Checking at other different recipes available, you will find that they suggest a 1:1 or 1:2 apple cider vinegar ratio without liquid.

I enjoy combining the liquid component with the vinegar part of apple cider and the steam part. Before pouring, don't forget to shake the apple cider vinegar, mainly if it's a natural ACV with the "mom" I was so happy about finally getting a smooth mixture when I first tested the straight mix. I drew a bath quickly, put on the mask, and sat down to relax. Within minutes of relaxing in the shower, my eyes began to water from the apple cider vinegar's strong scent. It didn't make a relaxing bath at all, so I found myself counting down the time until I was able to take off the damn thing. That's why I've been researching and suggesting combining the liquid component with part apple cider vinegar and part ice, and it's a much more fun overall experience.

I like apple cider vinegar, don't get me wrong. In reality, as my regular toner, I also use a diluted blend of ACV. Use undiluted apple cider vinegar directly on your body is not commonly recommended.

Water is entirely optional, blend one teaspoon of bentonite with two teaspoons of apple cider vinegar if you want to skip the water.

How to add Bentonite or Apple Cider Vinegar Mask to your face:

My favorite form for applying a mask is to use a facial mask comb. If you don't have one, you can add entirely with your hands.

By using a comb, you can stop adding bacteria to your skin that might be on your lips. For this reason, we put a brush in our facial clay mask multipack.

By applying my fingers, I also find that I lack material on my hands vs. using my face as much as I can.

Using the face mask brush to add the clay mask to my face gives me hallucinations to get a face where a mask is applied effortlessly by the esthetician and let me relax immediately.

Add an even surface to your mouth and jawline using the face mask comb. Don't get in your face too close or too near. Next, I like to add a thin layer on my head and then apply a second smaller layer.

You must add a mask coating of roughly 1/8'' to your body. So not a super thin application, but a medium one. It's going to look like below, and you can see how I put an excellent surface into it.

Ease Sunburn

Summer is here finally, and the sun's rays crank up their frequency as Mother Nature cranks up the mercury.

That's bound to lead to sunburn sooner or later. When you're out in the heat, it's always a good idea to wear sunscreen, but if you're burnt out, you're likely to be searching for a fast solution.

Due to its natural soothing properties, Aloe Vera is the typical go-to remedy, but there is another home remedy you may not have heard of: apple cider vinegar.

There are plenty of vinegar applications for apple cider. It is one of the most valuable brands that you can buy and is a natural alternative to a variety of household cleaners, personal care items, and medications.

The search for the ideal sun can go awry occasionally. This happens to the best of committed sun worshippers— too much time to soak up the sunlight and not enough sunscreen. If you do it on the beach or at the poolside and your skin feels like it's burning up, try using Apple Cider Vinegar (ACV) to relieve some of the pain and discomfort. Apple cider vinegar, when poured over the affected areas, absorbs warmth from sunburned skin. The scent of vinegar is not very good, but it will make your skin feel and look a lot better.

What Does Apple Cider Vinegar Do For Sunburn?

Apple cider vinegar is known for its ability to kill harmful bacteria while keeping good bacteria, according to the Wound Care Society.

Such effects tend to brighten up the sun as follows:

1.   Alleviating the sensation of pain and stinging.

2.   It is preventing inflammation of the body.

3.   It's Reduce the possibility of peeling, especially when accompanied by coconut oil.

Why Does Apple Cider Vinegar Help Sunburn?

Vinegar is a natural antiseptic that makes it ideal for the treatment of minor skin disorders such as slight rashes, eczema, and sunburn, of course. "Vinegar helps balance the pH (acid and alkalinity) of sunburned skin, facilitating regeneration, according to life-strong." Vinegar also reduces the likelihood that after burning the skin would develop blisters.

Apple Cider Vinegar Sunburn Remedy #1

The website of Butterbeliever advises the use of apple cider vinegar (ACV) to alleviate sunburn and replace it with coconut oil to moisturize the skin and avoid peeling. How to do it here:

1.   get a cold water warm washcloth.

2.   Splash any ACV and adhere to burnt skin on the damp washcloth.

3.   Achieve this by brushing the affected area with coconut oil.

Don't Go Back In The Sun If you're using this process, make sure that after adding coconut oil, you don't go back out in the sun. Research suggests that it provides almost no protection from the rays of the sun, contrary to popular belief.

Apple Cider Vinegar Sunburn Remedy #2

One way that you can use is an apple cider vinegar bath when the sun stings your hair. A simple method involves adding vinegar from apple cider to your tub and protecting your hair from sunburnt.

 Take the recommended procedures to take:

1.   Apply 2 cups of vinegar from apple cider to the bathwater. Water from the bathtub should not be cold, but cool.

2.   Thirty minutes in the tub.

3.   Protect the hair with a soft cotton towel by dabbing, not rubbing.

Apple Cider Vinegar Sunburn Remedy #3

Consider creating a soothing summer spritzer for severe sunburn in hard-to-reach places. To do this, dilute cold water apple cider vinegar and apply it to a bottle of spray. Then send a few quick showers to your skin whenever it starts heating up.

Here's a good sunburn cure with apple cider vinegar:

1.   Put 2 tbsps. Apple cider vinegar in a glass of water.

2.   In the same bottle, pour 1 cup of cold water.

3.   Shake the bottle and spray as necessary the affected area gently.

4.   Place the bottle for additional cooling relief in the fridge.

Insect Bites

The rains provide us with a much-needed respite from the scorching heat but at the cost of constant traffic jams, water pollution, asthma, and mosquito attacks. Welcome to the life of the town where there is still much more to contend with than enjoy. Mosquitoes are inevitable when it comes to enjoying the outdoors, particularly during the monsoons. This is a season of the full force of mosquitoes. You're going to have to agree, few things are as annoying as a bite of a mosquito and the itching, scratching and swelling it leads to. They bite you and feed on your blood and administer other chemicals that stop clotting of your blood, which triggers a slight allergic reaction, which leaves your skin sore, red bumps. Mosquito bites may be harmless, but they are itchy and can be painful at times. The good news is that you can get immediate relief, which takes just a little effort. You would be shocked to see how many things you will find in your kitchen that will help you fight the bite.

Directions

As soon as possible, add apple cider vinegar straight to the Vinegar bites–a small amount of apple cider vinegar can relieve the pain from the taste of a mosquito. In the alcohol, dip a cotton ball and keep on to the bite mark. You can also apply a few cups of vinegar to a tub if you have a lot of mosquito bites or drink until the itching subsides.

Apple Cider Vinegar is less acidic than other kinds of vinegar and tends to maintain healthy pH levels as well.

This is an excellent way of reducing sunburnt skin's pain and getting rid of redness.

Heal Bruise

Apple cider vinegar has anti-bacterial and anti-inflammatory qualities that have been used since ancient times for baking. Because it destroys bacteria and can be used as a cleaning agent, it is suitable for your skin, nutrition, hair, and even your home. The routine intake of ACV controls all of the internal body systems.

What's Bruises?

A bruise is a common skin discoloration that occurs after a traumatic injury from the breakage of tiny blood vessels bleeding under the body. Evidence from broken blood vessels under the skin pools near the surface to show as a black and blue sign that they remember. This mark is the result of red blood cells discoloring the skin and their contents. Sometimes known as a bruise is a wound.

What are bruises ' causes or risk factors?

People usually get body injuries when they run into something or when something bumps into it. Risk factors for bruises include:

• In some people who exercise rigorously, such as athletes and weight lifters, injuries can occur. Such marks are the result of small breaks in the under-skin blood vessels. Athlete bleeding can also be caused by direct impact/trauma or followed by an underlying hematoma (clotted blood).

• Unexplained, unexplained bruises that appear quickly or for no apparent reason can result in bleeding disorder or blood-thinning drugs (anticoagulants), mainly if frequent nosebleeds or bleeding gums follow the bruise.

• Sometimes, what are believed to be mysterious marks on the shine and leg, for example, are caused by bumps into a bedpost or other surface and fail to remember the accident.

•   Bruises frequently occur in the elderly due to thinner skin with age (senile purpura). It has become more delicate the structures that sustain the internal blood vessels.

•   Bruising on the back of the hands and arms (known as actinic purpura or solar purpura) happens because the skin is often thin or sun-damaged.

•   Vitamin C deficiency (ascorbic acid deficiency or scurvy) is more severe in bruises.

•   Bruising may be a symptom of the child's physical abuse (child abuse).

•   Alcohol abuse can make it easier for people to get hurt.

What are the causes or signs of a bruise?

•   The new bruise may be reddish in the middle. After a few hours, it will turn blue or dark purple, then yellow or green after a few days of healing.

•   For the first few days, a bruise is generally sore and sometimes even painful, but the pain usually goes away as the color disappears.

•   As they recover, bruises can itch.

•   There is little risk of infection because the skin is not split in a bruise like a scratch or a slice.

•   Repeated area bruising can leave permanent iron-depositing yellowish-brown staining in the skin.

•   Bruises typically last between one and two weeks, although some may take longer to heal.

How to use apple cider vinegar to heal wounds naturally.

1.   ACV can help reduce any irritation, swelling, or discomfort as it is a healthy anti-inflammatory. In a pan, add equal amounts of ACV and water. In this remedy, soak a paper towel and use it as a seal. Repeat till the swelling subsides every 20 minutes. If the skin is fractured or broken, do not follow this procedure.

2.   It is claimed that Apple cider vinegar increases blood flow after trauma, breaking up blood clots in damaged areas. It is typically dissolved and added as a seal of warm water.

Fade Bruise:

You can topically add apple cider vinegar to reduce the appearance of a bruise. Combine it with water and add it to the injury directly. Apply the concoction again once it has been cooled and try it 2-3 times. It will improve the bruise's discomfort, decrease redness, and boost the healing time as well.

Remove Warts:

Topically apply apple cider vinegar on the wart and then cover it with a band-aid or bandage. Leave overnight and take it out in the evening. You might see results in a week, or it might take longer. Apple cider vinegar has been claimed by thousands to heal warts and other skin problems.

Bee Sting Remedy:

Using apple cider vinegar to get bee sting relief quickly. Soak a ball of cotton in ACV and put it on the bite as soon as possible. Firstly it will hurt, but within a few minutes, you can feel relief. It will also stop nausea, and you'll also get rid of the pain. This cure has been used since ancient times and is very reliable.

Apple cider vinegar steam for sinus infection: Applying cider vinegar helps clear the sinus because of its Apply cider vinegar helps clear the sinus because of its anti-fungal, anti-bacterial, anti-inflammatory and immune-supporting effects, making it an excellent natural treatment for curing sinus infection. Get the cure here.

It is important to note that not all vinegar from apple cider is created equally! Make sure you buy it raw to get the most out of using ACV. The use of natural, unfiltered, and unpasteurized apple cider vinegar is imperative to reap both health and beauty benefits.

Nail fungus

We are asking a great deal from our foot. Throughout the day, we bear our bodies, often from uncomfortable shoes. It's no surprise that many of us end up with blisters, pressure, scent, and fungi, like the foot of an athlete.

Toenail fungus can be an unpleasant and persistent problem. Many of the over-the-counter drugs used to treat it are aggressive and often harmful, and prescription drugs can have severe side effects. That's why many toenail fungus patients are searching for a more effective and secure remedy. Apple cider vinegar is one of these therapies. It is organic, has fewer side effects, and it is far less costly than prescription or over-the-counter medications.

Fortunately, your woes have a simple solution, and it can be found in your kitchen.

Why vinegar?

Vinegar is a distilled, useful, and harmless source of acetic acid. We use it for cooking and cleaning — and healing our sore, weary, stinky feet.

According to one study, vinegar's antifungal effect is better than other meat preservatives, while being healthy enough to consume. It is this behavior that is blamed for some of its most significant advantages. Several forms of foot fungus have been found to slow the growth of vinegar.

Toenail Fungus Symptoms

 The Mayo Clinic reports typical toenail fungus symptoms such as thickened, brittle, crumbly and ragged toenails, toenail size change, dull-looking toenails, and toenail color darkening. If the infection is severe enough, the nail can be removed from the nail bed. Furthermore, the disease can cause some discomfort. Eventually, there may be a foul smell. Some or all of these symptoms may appear in an infected toenail. Early infection can appear in the tip of the nail as a small white or yellow mark.

Why Apple Cider Vinegar Works

The pH of the surrounding skin and nail becomes more alkaline and straightforward when a toenail fungus disease occurs. In a chemical climate, the fungus thrives. If the area's pH changes from basic to acidic, the fungus will not be able to survive. This is where it becomes useful for the apple cider vinegar. The vinegar is acidic but still mild that it does not harm the hair or nail around it.

Directions

Use apple cider vinegar as a toenail fungus remedy is one of the most common ways of using it as a foot bath. Livingclean's home remedy page recommends using a one-part vinegar and one-part air foot bath. The tub should have enough water to cover the feet fully. Using warm water for each other's foot bath for the most effective results. Some days, using cold water. Livingclean.com advises washing the feet for at least once a day for 30 minutes, but not more than three times a day. Upon withdrawing them from the tub, clean the feet thoroughly.

For athletes foot

Athlete's foot is a fungal infection affecting the toes for athlete's foot. The toes look red and may peel the hair. The foot of an athlete sometimes hurts or itches.

A vinegar soak can function well for mild forms of this disease. The antifungal effects also make the right choice for those with toenail fungus to drink vinegar. Soak your feet in a vinegar tub for 10 to 15 minutes a day until the disease is gone.

In the soak, you can gradually increase the length of time. Improvement of symptoms can take two to three weeks or longer. Better signs mean that the fungal disease has been treated long enough. Soaking your socks in vinegar may be a good idea, as well.

There are no tests of high quality that prove that vinegar is highly effective. Vinegar is not suitable for all forms of fungi, but in attempting this home treatment, there is little risk.

If the signs do not change, you should seek medical attention when they intensify and extend the foot. When you experience increased dryness and cracking, instead of regular, you may need to may your soaking to a few days a week.

For foot odor

Vinegar may also disinfect the feet for foot odor. Through getting rid of the bacteria that make them smell, it helps eliminate or reduce the scent of the foot.

Wash your feet properly with water and soap before soaking. Relax in a vinegar bath with your hands.

In addition to soaking, it is important to consider lifestyle choices when treating the odor of afoot. Consider, for example, wearing leather or canvas shoes. In comparison to shoes made from plastic materials, these allow your feet to breathe. Wear breathable socks of cotton and silk. Go barefoot when you're at work.

Quick tips

• Wear breathable socks of cotton and silk.

• Wear leather shoes or canvas that allow your feet to breathe.

• When you're at work, go barefoot.

For warts

Vinegar is a gentle exfoliator of moles, so you can use it to cure callous or warts as well. Upon bathing, you can use a pumice stone to file your feet and help you get rid of the hard skin. Vinegar can also be applied directly with a cotton ball to the affected areas.

For dry foots

Vinegar foot soaks will soothe hot, scratched feet with bare feet as well. Using cold water and wash the body with warm water. Soak at night before moisturizing the feet and slipping on shoes. Soaking too often or too long will make your feet drier, so use this soak sparingly for bare, broken feet.

Make the vinegar foot soak

Vinegar won't hurt your skin, but for a foot soak, you must dilute it. Usually, a reasonable balance is the use of 1-part vinegar to 2-part liquid. You can use a better soak if you accept the distilled vinegar soaks and do not notice any difference.

While the soak will smell heavy, after the vinegar dries from your feet, the scent will dissipate. You can also use essential oils to alter the smell slightly.

How to Use Apple Cider Vinegar

Without Soaking, Most people don't have the time to take two to three baths for 30 minutes a day. Another way to get the vinegar's results is to immediately add two drops of apple cider vinegar to the nail bed. Enable the vinegar to sit for several minutes on the nail bed without removing it or may not achieve the desired effect. This should be done twice a day at least. Together with the foot bath, this form can be used.

Treatment period

Such procedures must continue until all the infected nail has spread out and removed. Once a clean nail has replaced the diseased nail, any infection is unlikely to remain. This could take a few months or longer due to the slow growth of toenails. Clipping the infected nail regularly and keeping it clean and dry. After these treatments, it is necessary to dry the toenails thoroughly because the fungi like humid, hot, dark conditions. Since the toenails of each patient develop at a different rate, the actual treatment period can vary from person to person.

Caution

People with diabetes, peripheral vascular disease, or any other chronic condition affecting the flow of blood to the foot should be careful when trying to treat feet diseases. These conditions can cause the person to heal more slowly and become more susceptible to infection when a wound occurs on foot. Treatment should be performed under a trained health care professional's guidance. Vinegar can irritate the skin of the foot, according to the Mayo Clinic. The Mayo Clinic proposes two solutions to this problem: either lower the foot bath rate or use a higher proportion of water to dilute the vinegar. If the pain continues, interrupt the procedure and consult a doctor.

Vinegar is a cost-effective and easy-to-find cure for several foot problems. Not to mention, it can be refreshing to wash your feet after a long day.

Age Spots

Our bodies are evolving in unexpected ways as they age. We are beginning to notice the gray hairs and new aches and pains, and many are even seeing small brown spots all over our bodies.

Black spots are also known as freckles, sunspots, age spots, and so on and are caused by excess skin exposure to the sun, zits, wrinkles, blemishes, and blackheads. Most of the time, dark spots are caused by acne or wounds that leave behind scars that may also seem dark. Apple cider vinegar is an all-rounder hair booster with many skin advantages like lighting up the face and body with dark spots.

Why can't vinegar apple cider do? The cheap pantry staple softens hair, helps control the production of oil and acne, and it has been established (drumroll, please) to lighten dark spots. This succeeds because it accelerates the process of skin removal and regrowth, which, of course, means adding a new skin to the surface earlier, which is not discolored.

Here's how to get rid of dark spots using apple cider vinegar:

Onion + apple cider vinegar

Onions help remove scars and places related to acne. Break an onion into several pieces, roast them and extract the juice from the crushed onions. Combine it in (equal quantities) with apple cider vinegar and add this mixture to the affected areas of the skin; permit the combination to stay overnight. Wash the day clean.

Turmeric + apple cider vinegar

Turmeric is a skin-illuminating agent that can also be used to get rid of black spots on your body. Create a thick paste with vinegar with turmeric or apple cider. Apply it to the skin where black spots are present. Keep it on for 30 minutes, then rinse it with tippy steam.

Buttermilk + apple cider vinegar

Buttermilk is known for its bleaching properties, which helps to make dark spots darker and rid them. Mix buttermilk and apple cider vinegar in equal quantities and use it as a face mask. Upon 10 minutes of cleaning. Instead, in apple cider vinegar, you can mix sugar to form a paste and use it as a face scrub. Between 5-10 minutes, rinse with air to see the desired results.

Note: Always do an allergic reaction patch test.

Cure Acne

For your digestive system, Apple cider vinegar is good. But do you know that when it comes to making acne disappear, it works like magic? Indeed! ACV is one of Nature's most effective weapons for healing most (especially acne) skin-related woes. If you still ask how and why ACV works for acne, let's take a closer look at Is

Apple Cider Vinegar Great for Acne

Not enough research has been done to show that ACV tends to treat acne. Nevertheless, the good news is, we've collected some evidence that shows it might help battle acne-causing bacteria.

For destroying several strains of bacteria, vinegar is beneficial. While there are not many studies showing that apple cider vinegar can kill the bacterial strain that causes acne, this can be achieved by the organic compounds present in the vinegar. Let's look at it:

1. It Kills The Acne-Causing Bacteria

Two independent studies published in Applied Microbiology and Biotechnology and International Journal of Cosmetic Science suggest that acetic acid, lactic acid, citric acid, and succinic acids can destroy Propionibacterium acnes or P. acnes, the bacteria that cause acne. And all these acids are contained in apple cider vinegar.

2. It Helps Reduce Acne

Another study published in the Indian Journal of Dermatology, Venereology, and Leprology found that people who applied a lotion containing lactic acid to their heads had a reduction in their acne. The vinegar in apple cider also contains lactic acid.

3. It Reduces Scars

It may help to reduce the scars left behind once the acne is cured by Marks Apple cider vinegar. In this process, many organic compounds assist. The process is called chemical peeling if you add acid straight to your head. Chemical peeling suppresses inflammation caused by acne when performed with succinic acid. It helps to avoid scarring.

Also, lactic acid helps those with acne's skin condition. With all these acids in apple cider vinegar, we can expect promising results.

Let's now take a detailed look at how you can cure acne with apple cider vinegar on your face.

Tips To Use Apple Cider Vinegar For Acne

ACV can be used in two ways:

(I) apply topically (mix it in your face pack and add the condensed form directly to your skin).

(ii) Remove the morning coffee with a tablespoon.

All the ways you can include apple cider vinegar in your daily beauty and wellness regimen to reduce acne are listed below.

Ways To Get Rid Of Acne With Topical Application Of Apple Cider Vinegar

1. Apple Cider Vinegar Toner For Acne

Ingredients

•	Two teaspoons of apple cider vinegar (organic with mother)

•	2 cups of water

•	One teaspoon aloe vera gel

Preparation

• Blend both ingredients.

• In a spray bottle, hold the solution.

How can I apply

1. Sprinkle the toner gently around your face and neck.

How does it work

Aloe Vera gel has anti-inflammatory effects and soothes the skin. Apple cider vinegar's astringent properties kill the bacteria that cause acne and reduce inflammation. This toner can also be used for back acne. It is appropriate for all forms of hair.

Precaution

Close your eyes while spraying to stop the toner from slipping into them. Do not use it on dried or fractured skin as well.

Ingredients

• Two tablespoons of apple cider vinegar

• Three tablespoons of baking soda

Preparation

• Blend the baking soda with the apple cider vinegar in a small bowl.

How to use

1.   Attach the mask to the area in question.

2.   Keep it on and rinse it off for 20 minutes.

3.   Use a moisturizer to suit this.

How does it work

Baking soda also has anti-inflammatory effects that help reduce skin inflammation, along with apple cider vinegar. This exfoliates the body, unblocks the pores, eliminates the cells that are debris and dead, and preserves the skin's pH level.

Precaution

Baking soda does not fit all forms of hair. Do a patch test if you have sensitive skin. Avoid using it in the event of scratching or swelling of the body.

Conclusion

Recently apple cider vinegar has been deemed a very helpful health elixir. What once used to be considered folk remedies using this is now backed by scientific research indicating its helpful effects. The primary ingredient is acetic acid. Vinegars also have other acids, vitamins, mineral salts and amino acids.

Vinegar is a product of the process of fermentation by which sugars in a food are broken down by bacteria in yeast. In the second stage of fermentation the alcohol ferments further and we get vinegar. Specifically, apple cider vinegar comes from crushed apples.

Because of the widespread claims that it can promote health benefits, scientific evidence has been evaluated and has shown that this indeed is true.

The popularity of apple cider vinegar continues to this day. And the best part is that it is readily available at your local supermarket.

TRY APPLE CIDER VINEGAR TODAY!

www.ingramcontent.com/pod-product-compliance
Lightning Source LLC
Chambersburg PA
CBHW060326030426
42336CB00011B/1217